Comprehensive Manuals of Surgical Specialties

Richard H. Egdahl, editor

Manual of Sports Surgery

Kerlan-Jobe Orthopaedic Clinic

Edited by
Clarence L. Shields, Jr.

With Contributions by Clive E. Brewster, Vincent S. Carter
H. Royer Collins, Robert K. Kerlan, Stephen J. Lombardo
Matthew C. Morrissey, Judy L. Seto, Clarence L. Shields, Jr.
James E. Tibone, Lewis A. Yocum

Illustrated by Robin Markovits Jensen

Includes 257 Illustrations, 139 in Full Color

Springer-Verlag
New York Berlin Heidelberg
London Paris Tokyo

SERIES EDITOR

Richard H. Egdahl, M.D., Ph.D., Professor of Surgery, Boston University Medical Center, Boston, Massachusetts 02118, USA

EDITOR

Clarence L. Shields Jr, M.D., Kerlan-Jobe Orthopaedic Clinic, Inglewood, California 90301, USA

DEVELOPMENTAL EDITOR

Martin S. Stanford, Brooklyn, New York 11215, USA

MEDICAL ILLUSTRATOR

Robin Markovits Jensen, M.S.M.I., Portland, Oregon 97201, USA

Library of Congress Cataloging in Publication Data
Manual of sports surgery.
   (Comprehensive manuals of surgical specialties)
   Includes bibliographies and index.
   1. Sports—Accidents and injuries—Handbooks,
manuals, etc.   2. Sports medicine—Handbooks,
manuals, etc.   3. Surgery—Handbooks, manuals, etc.
I. Shields, Clarence L., Jr.   II. Brewster, Clive E.
III. Series.   [DNLM: 1. Sports Medicine.
2. Surgery, QT 260 M294]
RD97.M36   1987   617'.1027   86–22631

Typeset by Arcata Graphics/Kingsport, Kingsport, Tennessee.
Printed and bound by Universitätsdruckerei Stürtz AG, Würzburg, Federal Republic of Germany.
Printed in the Federal Republic of Germany.

9 8 7 6 5 4 3 2 1

ISBN 0-387-96415-0 Springer-Verlag New York Berlin Heidelberg
ISBN 3-540-96415-0 Springer-Verlag Berlin Heidelberg New York

Editor's Note

Comprehensive Manuals of Surgical Specialties is a series of surgical manuals designed to present current operative techniques and to explore various aspects of diagnosis and treatment. The series features a unique format with emphasis on large, detailed, full-color illustrations, schematic charts, and photographs to demonstrate integral steps in surgical procedures.

Each manual focuses on a specific region or topic and describes surgical anatomy, physiology, pathology, diagnosis, and operative treatment. Operative techniques and stratagems for dealing with surgically correctable disorders are described in detail. Illustrations are primarily depicted from the surgeon's viewpoint to enhance clarity and comprehension.

Other volumes in the series:

Published:

Manual of Burns
Manual of Surgery of the Gallbladder, Bile Ducts,
*   and Exocrine Pancreas*
Manual of Urologic Surgery
Manual of Lower Gastrointestinal Surgery
Manual of Vascular Surgery, Volume I
Manual of Vascular Surgery, Volume II
Manual of Cardiac Surgery, Volume I
Manual of Cardiac Surgery, Volume II
Manual of Liver Surgery
Manual of Ambulatory Surgery
Manual of Pulmonary Surgery
Manual of Soft-Tissue Tumor Surgery
Manual of Endocrine Surgery (Second Edition)
Manual of Vascular Access, Organ Donation,
*   and Transplantation*
Manual of Aesthetic Surgery
Manual of Upper Gastrointestinal Surgery
Manual of Gynecologic Surgery (Second Edition)

vi

In Preparation:

Manual of Orthopedic Surgery
Manual of Trauma Surgery
Manual of Reconstructive Surgery
Manual of Urologic Surgery (Second Edition)

Richard H. Egdahl

Foreword

This manual presents the operations most often performed by surgeons at the Kerlan-Jobe Orthopaedic Clinic (Inglewood, California, 90301) in treating sports injuries. These operations constitute a complete series of basic surgical procedures for the orthopaedist. In its step-by-step drawings, the manual guides surgeons through the operative techniques of specific procedures. It also provides what is equally important for practitioners: the protocols for postoperative care of patients, including the rehabilitation of those who have—and have not—had to undergo surgery.

It must also be said that this manual is not a be-all and end-all of surgical interventions and rehabilitative programs for athletes, amateur or professional, who sustain injuries on the playing field. That elusive goal can only be reached by practitioners who attend strictly to all the diagnostic detail available, who select carefully those patients most likely to benefit from their attention and care, and who share with other practitioners their experience and expertise.

As far as diagnosis is concerned, there has been a great improvement in the recent past in both noninvasive and invasive procedures that help to establish specific diagnoses and to determine which patients will be served best by a given operation. These new diagnostic tools include the arthrogram in conjunction with the tomogram and the CT scan; the CT scan itself; the arthroscope; and, most recently, the Magnetic Resonance Imaging machine.

As far as the patients themselves are concerned, this manual is based on a fundamental premise: patients are not objects to be diagnosed, operated on, and rehabilitated. Instead, they are individual persons who are sensitively and intimately concerned about their own respective conditions. The surgeon must recognize and understand their varying psychological tendencies so that he may be a caring physician in the fullest sense of the term rather than a well-wired and efficiently programmed robot.

Robert K. Kerlan, M.D.

Acknowledgments

I would like to thank the administration of Centinela Hospital Medical Center for their encouragement and support during this project. I wish to express my most sincere appreciation in the development of this book to the medical library staff as well as the staff of the medical photography department at Centinela Hospital Medical Center. I would like to give a special thanks to my secretary, Cindy Covington, for her time and efforts.

Contents

Editor's Note by Richard H. Egdahl   v
Foreword by Robert K. Kerlan   vii
Acknowledgment   viii
Contributors   xvii

I Shoulder

1 Arthroscopy   2
Stephen J. Lombardo

   General Considerations   2
   Surgical Procedure and Techniques   2
References   7
Additional Reading   7

2 Impingement Syndrome   8
H. Royer Collins, Vincent S. Carter, and
Clarence L. Shields, Jr.

Coracoacromial Ligament Resection   8
   General Considerations   8
   Surgical Procedure and Techniques   9
   Postoperative Care and Rehabilitation   10
Rotator Cuff Repair   11
   General Considerations   11
   Surgical Procedure and Techniques   11
   Postoperative Care and Rehabilitation   16
Bicipital Tenodesis   16
   General Considerations   16
   Surgical Procedure and Techniques   17

References   19
Additional Reading   19

3   Anterior Reconstruction   20
Stephen J. Lombardo

Modified Bristow Procedure   20
    General Considerations   20
    Surgical Procedure and Techniques   20
    Postoperative Care and Rehabilitation   27
Anterior Staple Capsulorrhaphy   27
    General Considerations   27
    Surgical Procedure and Techniques   27
References   30
Additional Reading   30

4   Posterior Reconstruction   32
James E. Tibone

    General Considerations   32
    Surgical Procedure and Techniques   32
    Postoperative Care and Rehabilitation   36
References   37
Additional Reading   37

II   Elbow

5   Arthroscopy   40
Lewis A. Yocum

    General Considerations   40
    Surgical Procedure and Techniques   40
References   42
Additional Reading   42

6   Lateral Epicondyle Release   43
H. Royer Collins

    General Considerations   43
    Surgical Procedure and Techniques   43
    Postoperative Care and Rehabilitation   45

References 45
Additional Reading 45

7 Debridement 46
James E. Tibone and H. Royer Collins

General Considerations 46
Surgical Procedure and Techniques 46
Postoperative Care and Rehabilitation 48
References 48
Additional Reading 48

8 Medial Collateral Ligament Reconstruction 49
H. Royer Collins and Clarence L. Shields, Jr.

General Considerations 49
Surgical Procedure and Techniques 49
Postoperative Care and Rehabilitation 52
References 52
Additional Reading 52

9 Ulnar Nerve Transfer 53
H. Royer Collins

General Considerations 53
Surgical Procedure and Techniques 53
Postoperative Care and Rehabilitation 55
References 55
Additional Reading 56

10 Repair of Distal Biceps Tendon Rupture 57
James E. Tibone

General Considerations 57
Surgical Procedure and Techniques 57
Postoperative Care and Rehabilitation 61
References 61
Additional Reading 61

11 Rehabilitation of the Upper Extremity 62

Clive E. Brewster, Clarence L. Shields, Jr., Judy L. Seto, and Matthew C. Morrissey

Determining Rehabilitative Goals 62
Basic Rehabilitation Protocol: The Shoulder 62
Special Rehabilitation Protocols: The Shoulder 82
Basic Rehabilitation Protocol—The Elbow 84
References 89
Additional Reading 89

III Knee

12 Arthroscopy 92

Lewis A. Yocum

General Considerations 92
Surgical Procedure and Techniques 92
References 98
Additional Reading 98

13 Patellar Malalignment Syndromes 99

Clarence L. Shields, Jr.

General Considerations 99
Surgical Procedure and Techniques 100
Postoperative Care and Rehabilitation 104
References 104
Additional Reading 104

14 Repair of Extensor Mechanism Injuries 105

Clarence L. Shields, Jr.

General Considerations 105
Patellar Tendinitis Repair 105
Surgical Procedure and Techniques 105
Postoperative Care and Rehabilitation 106
Repair of Patellar Tendon Rupture 107
Surgical Procedure and Techniques 107
Postoperative Care and Rehabilitation 109

References   109
Additional Reading   110

15 Repair of Medial Collateral Ligament (MCL) Injuries   111
H. Royer Collins and Clarence L. Shields, Jr.

Acute MCL (Including Cruciate Ligament) Repair   111
   General Considerations   111
   Surgical Procedure and Techniques   112
   Postoperative Care and Rehabilitation   118
Chronic MCL Repair   119
   General Considerations   119
   Surgical Procedure and Techniques   119
   Postoperative Care and Rehabilitation   120
References   121
Additional Reading   121

16 Repair of Lateral Collateral Ligament (LCL) Injuries   123
H. Royer Collins and Clarence L. Shields, Jr.

Acute LCL Repair   123
   General Considerations   123
   Surgical Procedure and Techniques   123
   Postoperative Care and Rehabilitation   125
Chronic LCL Repair   125
   General Considerations   125
   Surgical Procedure and Techniques   126
   Postoperative Care and Rehabilitation   127
References   127
Additional Reading   127

17 Repair of Posterior Cruciate Ligament (PCL) Injuries   128
H. Royer Collins and Clarence L. Shields, Jr.

Acute PCL Repair   128
   General Considerations   128
   Surgical Procedure and Techniques   128
Chronic PCL Repair   129
   General Considerations   129
   Surgical Procedure and Techniques   130
   Postoperative Care and Rehabilitation   133

References 133
Additional Reading 133

18 Repair of Chronic Anterior Cruciate Ligament (ACL) Injuries 134
Clarence L. Shields, Jr.

General Considerations 134
Pes Anserinus Transfer 135
  Surgical Procedure or Techniques 135
Ellison Procedure 138
  Surgical Procedure and Techniques 138
Intra-Articular Patellar Tendon Transfer 142
  Surgical Procedure and Techniques 142
  Postoperative Care and Rehabilitation 147
References 148
Additional Reading 148

IV Ankle

19 Arthroscopy 152
Lewis A. Yocum

General Considerations 152
Surgical Procedure and Techniques 152
References 154
Additional Reading 154

20 Repair of Achilles Tendon Injuries 155
Clarence L. Shields, Jr.

Tendinitis and Partial Rupture Repair 155
  General Considerations 155
  Postoperative Recovery and Rehabilitation 158
Complete Rupture Repair 158
  General Considerations 158
  Surgical Procedure and Techniques 158
  Postoperative Recovery and Rehabilitation 160
References 161
Additional Reading 161

21 Repair of Chronic Lateral Ligament
Injuries   162
Lewis A. Yocum

Brostrom Procedure for Reconstruction   162
    General Considerations   162
    Surgical Procedure and Techniques   162
    Postoperative Recovery and Rehabilitation   165
Chrisman-Snook Procedure for Reconstruction   165
    General Considerations   165
    Surgical Procedure and Techniques   166
    Postoperative Care and Rehabilitation   169
References   169
Additional Reading   169

22 Treatment of Osteochondritis
Dissecans of the Talus   171
Lewis A. Yocum

    General Considerations   171
    Surgical Procedure and Techniques   171
    Postoperative Recovery and Rehabilitation   173
References   175
Additional Reading   175

23 Rehabilitation of the Lower
Extremity   176
Clarence L. Shields, Jr., Clive E. Brewster, and
Matthew C. Morrissey

    Immediate Postoperative Rehabilitation   176
    Determining Rehabilitative Goals   177
    Basic Rehabilitation Protocol: The Knee   178
    Rehabilitation Protocols: Special Conditions   189
References   198
Additional Reading   200

Index   201

Contributors

Clive E. Brewster, M.S., R.P.T., Director of Physical Therapy, Kerlan-Jobe Orthopaedic Clinic, Inglewood, California

Vincent S. Carter, M.D., Associate Professor, Clinical Emergency Medicine, University of Southern California School of Medicine, Los Angeles, California

H. Royer Collins, M.D., Institute for Bone and Joint Disorders, Phoenix, Arizona

Robert K. Kerlan, M.D., Clinical Professor of Orthopaedics, University of Southern California School of Medicine; Orthopaedic Consultant to Los Angeles Lakers, Los Angeles Rams, California Angels; Kerlan-Jobe Orthopaedic Clinic, Inglewood, California

Stephen J. Lombardo, M.D., Clinical Associate Professor of Orthopaedics, University of Southern California School of Medicine; Orthopaedic Surgeon Sports Medicine; Team Physician to Los Angeles Lakers, Los Angeles Kings; Kerlan-Jobe Orthopaedic Clinic, Inglewood, California

Matthew C. Morrissey, M.A., P.T., Assistant Professor, Department of Physical Therapy, University of Wisconsin-La Crosse, La Crosse, Wisconsin

Judy L. Seto, M.A., P.T., Coordinator of Physical Therapy Research, Department of Physical Therapy, Kerlan-Jobe Orthopaedic Clinic, Inglewood, California

Clarence L. Shields, Jr., M.D., Clinical Assistant Professor of Orthopaedics, University of Southern California School of Medicine; Clinical Assistant Professor, Charles Drew School of Medicine, Los Angeles California; Orthopaedic Surgeon Sports Medicine; Team Physician to Los Angeles Rams; Orthopaedic Consultant to Los Angeles Lakers, Los Angeles Dodgers, Los Angeles Kings, California Angels; Kerlan-Jobe Orthopaedic Clinic, Inglewood, California

James E. Tibone, M.D., Clinical Assistant Professor of Orthopaedic Surgery, University of Southern California School of Medicine, Los Angeles, California; Team Physician to Los Angeles Kings, Los Angeles Lakers

Lewis A. Yocum, M.D., Clinical Assistant Professor of Orthopaedics, University of Southern California School of Medicine, Los Angeles, California; Orthopaedic Surgeon, Sports Medicine; Team Physician to California Angels; Director of Sports Injury Clinic, Centinela Hospital Medical Center

Shoulder

I

1 Arthroscopy

Stephen J. Lombardo

General Considerations

The most commonly arthroscoped joint in the body, excluding the knee, is the shoulder.[1-4] Shoulder joint arthroscopy is indicated whenever:

1. The patient presents with persistent, undiagnosed pain that does not respond to conservative measures over an adequate period of time.
2. The patient reports repetitive episodes of "locking" crepitus and subluxation that examination fails to document and that conservative management fails to lessen in frequency and severity.
3. The physician suspects any of the following conditions: rotator cuff tear not documented by arthrogram; partial biceps tendon rupture; labral or osteochondral lesions, including loose bodies; chondromalacia; old fracture; Bankart, reverse Bankart, or Hill-Sachs lesions; unidirectional or multidirectional instability.

Surgical Procedure and Techniques

Perform the following procedure under general anesthesia while the patient is in a lateral decubitus position with the affected shoulder uppermost. First, maintain the patient's position with either Olympic Vac-Pac Surgical Positioning System "bean bag" or chest supports so that the shoulder can be prepped and draped free to permit a full arc of motion during the procedure. Either a pulley system with Buck's traction can be applied to the forearm or a commercial traction setup can be utilized. Next, abduct the extremity 40 to 60 degrees (Fig. 1-1A) and flex it forward 10 to 20 degrees (Fig. 1-1B); then, if you have chosen a pulley system, add weights of 5 to 15 pounds. In doing so, be sure to remove the weight every 30 minutes for 5- to 10-minute intervals to help avoid neurovascular complications.

The posterolateral corner of the acromion and the coracoid process anteriorly are two important anatomic landmarks for insertion of the arthroscope. The neurovascular structures posteriorly are the suprascapular nerve, which is located superomedial, and the axillary nerve, which is inferolateral to the point of entry of the instruments. Superiorly, the suprascapular nerve enters through the suprascapular notch, which is about 5 cm from the posterior portal of insertion; 5 to 6 cm inferiorly, the axillary nerve is located at the quadrangular space (Fig. 1-2A).

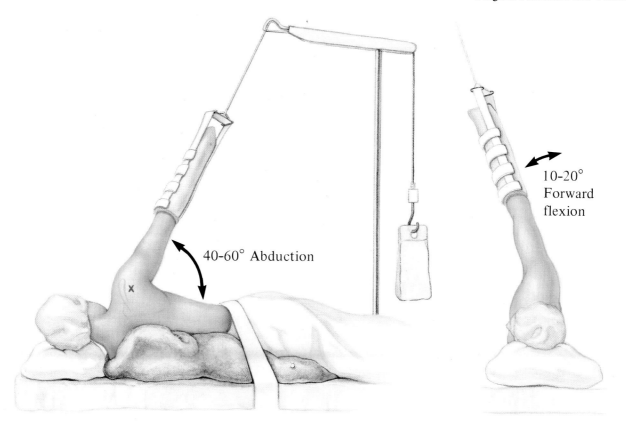

FIGURE 1-1A. Abduction.   FIGURE 1-1B. Forward flexion.

Using a 21-gauge spinal needle, inject the joint with normal saline to distend it. Insert the needle 2 to 3 cm inferior and 2 to 3 cm medial to the posterolateral corner of the acromion. Direct the needle toward the palpable anterior coracoid process (Fig. 1-2B), which is parallel to the plane of the anterior slope of the glenoid.

When the pulley system is used and the arm is suspended, determine the position of the needle as follows. If the needle touches the head of the humerus—as it is intended to—there will be a slight reactive motion of the arm; if, instead, the needle comes into contact with the stable glenoid or scapula neck, there will be no visible reactive motion. The usual course of the needle is through the middle of the infraspinatus tendon, slightly medial to its capsular insertion at the greater tuberosity of the humerus. Up to 50 ml of normal saline can be infused into the joint, although this capacity may be restricted if a patient presents with adhesive capsulitis. Once the fluid is infused, remove the needle. Prior to making a 1 to 1.5 cm incision with a #11 blade for insertion of the arthroscope, infiltrate posteriorly along the same needle track 2 to 3 ml of 0.25 percent bupavicaine (Marcaine) with epinephrine 1:200,000.

The arthroscope can vary from 2.7 to 5.0 mm in diameter; however, arthroscopes of 4.0 to 5.0 mm permit better visualization. (I prefer a 4.0 mm arthroscope for maximum visualization. Under these conditions, the entire joint can be seen.)

Gentle distraction of the joint at 30 to 60 degrees of abduction may facilitate insertion of the obturator with trocar. Ideally, one should enter the capsule with a sharp trocar and the synovium with a blunt trocar. When the joint is entered, a palpable thrust can be discerned. If a cloudy or bloody fluid is encountered, insert an egress needle anteriorly.

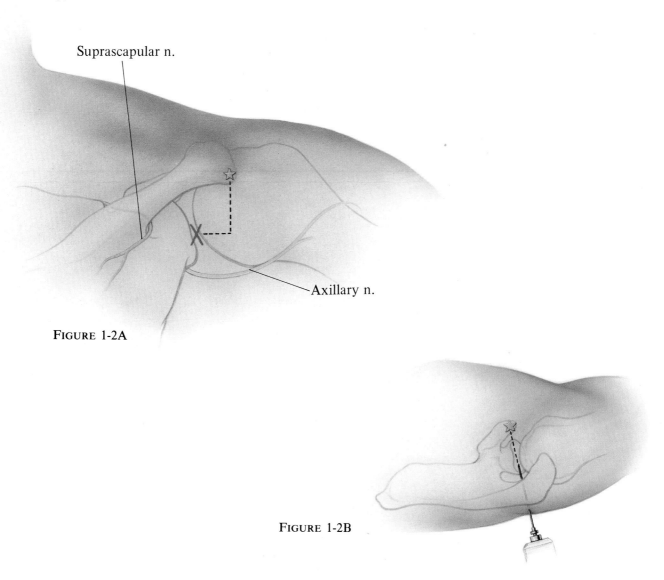

Suprascapular n.

Axillary n.

FIGURE 1-2A

FIGURE 1-2B

By taking a posterior approach, with the arthroscope, you can visualize the superior, middle, and inferior aspects of the joint, both anterior and posteriorly (Fig. 1-3). The anatomic structures that can be seen include biceps tendon, glenohumeral ligaments, glenoid and labrum, humeral head, and rotator cuff. By changing the degrees of distraction, forward flexion, abduction, and rotation of the arm, access to certain parts of the joint become easier.

Alternate Portals

Initially I prefer to insert the arthroscope posteriorly; then under direct vision, insert the instruments anteriorly. The light of the posterior-positioned arthroscope, when pressed anteriorly, can be used as a guide for insertion of the instruments (Fig. 1-4).

The presence of the cephalic vein and of the biceps tendon in the region of the deltopectoral groove increases the potential for complications. For this reason, insert the instruments approximately 2 to 4 cm lateral and superior to the coracoid process after rotating the arm externally. First, however, I usually insert anteriorly a 21-gauge spinal needle in order to be sure that the tract being used will not violate the biceps tendon. Prior to inserting the instruments, inject Marcaine with epinephrine into the subcutaneous tissue. To facilitate the exchange of instruments, insert a cannula.

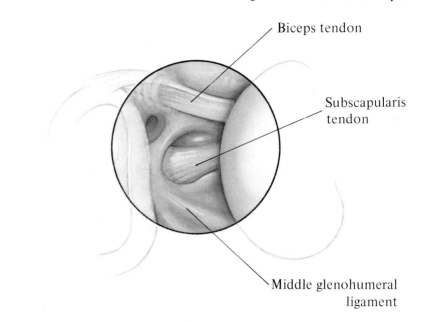

Biceps tendon

Subscapularis
tendon

Middle glenohumeral
ligament

FIGURE 1-3.   Posterior portal view.

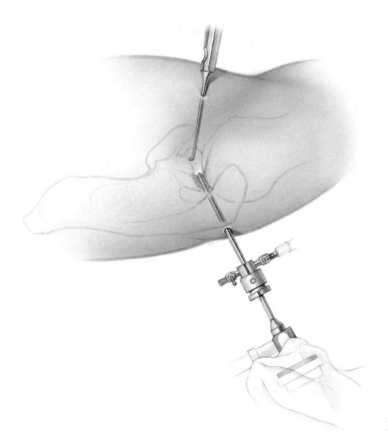

FIGURE 1-4.   Posterior portal.

To insert an arthroscope anteriorly, introduce a rod through the cannula
of the posterior-positioned arthroscope. By directing the rod anteriorly and
pressing it against the anterior structures, the skin will begin to tent (Fig.
1-5). A small incision over this area will then permit the rod to be pushed
through the skin. Once this is done, insert an anterior arthroscope over this
rod. The scope penetrates between the subscapularis muscle and biceps tendon
(Fig. 1-6A, 6B). A third portal can then be used anterior or posterior, superior
or interior, to the initial portal. Insert a cannula for the draining of fluids

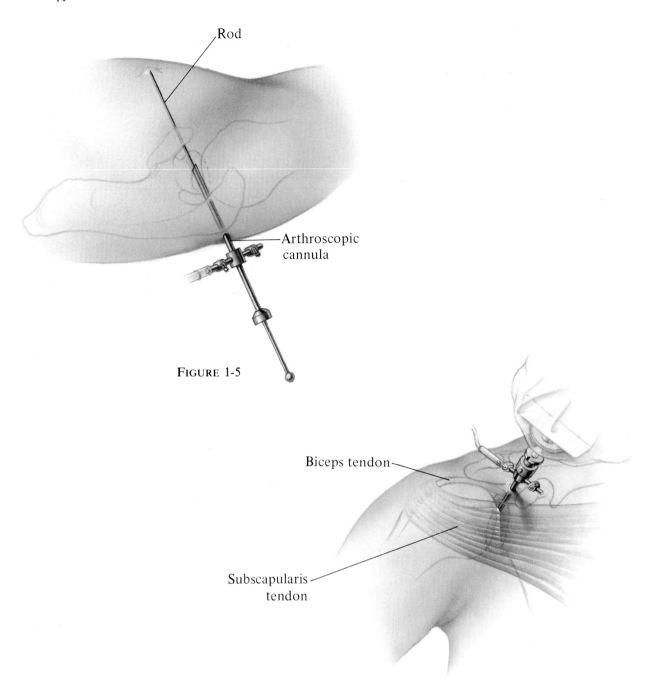

Rod

Arthroscopic
cannula

FIGURE 1-5

Biceps tendon

Subscapularis
tendon

FIGURE 1-6A.   Anterior portal.

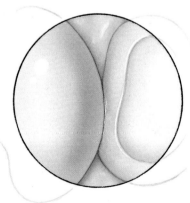

FIGURE 1-6B.   Anterior portal view.

or the passing of other instruments. The fluid egress needle may be inserted slightly medial to the junction of the clavicle and acromion and then directed from a superior medial position to an inferior lateral direction through the rotator cuff.

Operative Arthroscopy

The principal surgery done transarthroscopically is to excise or debride labral lesions, to remove loose bodies, and to excise tissue for biopsies. Occasionally, other surgical procedures can also be performed: debridement of fragments of the biceps tendon and rotator cuff; chondroplasty with certain articular cartilage lesions; and, when indicated, synovectomy (e.g., in the knee). At present, staple capsulorrhaphy for instability is only in the investigative stage. Strict adherence to aseptic conditions and proper orientation and technique will help avoid neurovascular and infectious problems.

References

1. Johnson LL: Arthroscopy of the shoulder. *Orthop Clin North Am* 1980;11:197–204.
2. Johnson LL: *Diagnostic and Surgical Arthroscopy,* 2nd ed. St. Louis, Mosby, 1981, pp. 376–389.
3. Wiley AM, Older MWJ: Shoulder arthroscopy, investigations with a fibro-optic instrument. *Am J Sports Med* 1980;8:31–38.
4. Lombardo SJ: Arthroscopy of the shoulder. *Clin Sports Med* 1983;2:309–318.

Additional Reading

Andrews JR, Carson WG, Ortega K: Arthroscopy of the shoulder: Technique and normal anatomy. *Am J Sports Med* 1984;12:1–7.

Johnson LL: Arthroscopy of the shoulder. *Orthop Clin North Am* 1980;11:197–204.

Lilleby H: Shoulder arthroscopy. *Acta Orthop Scand* 1984; 55:561–566.

McGlynn FJ, Caspari RB: Arthroscopic findings in the subluxating shoulder. *Clin Orthop* 1984;183:173–178.

Parisien JS: Shoulder arthroscopy: Technique and indications. *Bull Hosp Jt Dis Orthop Inst* 1983;43:56–69.

2 Impingement Syndrome

H. Royer Collins, Vincent S. Carter, and
Clarence L. Shields, Jr.

Coracoacromial Ligament Resection

General Considerations

Patients who present with impingement syndrome of the shoulder and have
not responded to the usual conservative measures are often candidates for
resection of the coracoacromial ligament.[1] This procedure is most successful
when carried out on patients who show the following characteristics: (1) are
under the age of 30; and (2) have the following kind of history. Initially,
the shoulder symptoms of these patients respond to conservative measures
(e.g., nonsteroidal anti-inflammatory agents, rest, ice, and other physical therapy modalities as well as a good exercise program and/or injections of steroids).
Subsequently, however, these patients re-present with the original symptoms
whenever they go back to the activities that produced the impingement syndrome in the first place. Such activities are swimming, pitching, serving in
tennis, weight lifting (particularly military press), and other activities that
require a motion of the shoulder greater than 90 degrees of abduction. In
these instances, the rotator cuff and/or the biceps tendon with the overlying
bursa impinge under the coracoacromial ligament to produce friction and
cause irritation of these structures.[2]

The diagnosis of impingement syndrome is made by a history of certain
kinds of activities. These repetitive overhead motions, as mentioned, become
unremittingly painful and eventually lead to difficulty in sleeping and in bringing the arm through a full range of motion.[3] The pain is produced when
the shoulder is brought through an arc of motion from 70 to about 110
degrees. Frequently, once the structures of the rotator cuff, biceps tendon,
and the bursa have moved out from under the coracoacromial arch, the pain
is no longer present. This usually occurs once the arm is abducted beyond
110 degrees.

Care must be taken to differentiate between pain coming from the acromioclavicular joint and that coming from subluxation of the shoulder. A history
of injury to the shoulder, such as a fall on the point of the shoulder or on
the outstretched arm, should alert the physician to either of these two possibili-
ties. If the patient is asked to touch the opposite shoulder with the hand of
the involved arm, the humerus will be brought into adduction and the symp-

8

toms accentuated from the acromioclavicular joint. If there is also bicipital tendinitis, there may be tenderness along the biceps groove. And, if some degenerative change is occurring in the supraspinatus muscle, there will be weakness with the arm held out in abduction and flexed forward 20 degrees.[4]

Although resection of the coracoacromial ligament is a simple procedure in itself, it is often unsuccessful when used on a patient over 30 years of age because there may be some osteophyte formation underneath the acromion. In the older patient, the resection must be combined with an acromioplasty to remove the osteophytes. (See the following section on rotator cuff repair.) This procedure is also contraindicated where there is extensive degenerative arthritis of the shoulder joint.

Surgical Procedure and Techniques

The procedure is usually carried out with the patient under general anesthesia in a supine position. Place the patient in a semisitting position on the operating table. I prefer not to use a sandbag under the shoulder because it tends to protract the shoulder and make it a little more difficult to expose the coracoacromial (CA) ligament through the small incision that is used. After the usual prepping and draping and with the arm draped free, extend an incision for 2 cm from the acromioclavicular (A-C) joint distally in line with the lines of Langerhans (Fig. 2-1). At this point, use small rake retractors to expose the anterior deltoid muscle. Next, split the deltoid in line with its fibers for a distance of approximately 1 cm distally from the A-C joint (Fig. 2-2). Use scissor dissection to open this interval and expose the coracoacromial ligament with a Kocher's clamp to delineate it. Once this is accomplished, the entire extent of the coracoacromial ligament can be delineated.

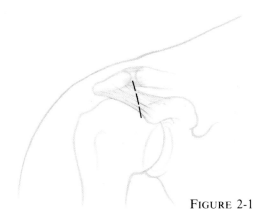

FIGURE 2-1

Using a #15 blade scalpel, resect the coracoacromial ligament from its coracoid tip and then from its attachment under the acromion (Fig. 2-3). Take care that all of the ligament is exposed, but be aware while doing so that the branches of the acromial artery lie under the clavicle and may cause troublesome bleeding if they are cut during removal of the ligament.

Once the ligament is removed, the subacromial bursa is apparent. At this point, note whether the bursa is excessively thickened and inflamed and thus requires excision. The biceps tendon can also be visualized through this incision and any pathology noted. Stop all bleeding and allow the fibers of the deltoid muscle to fall back into place after thoroughly irrigating the wound with sterile saline solution.

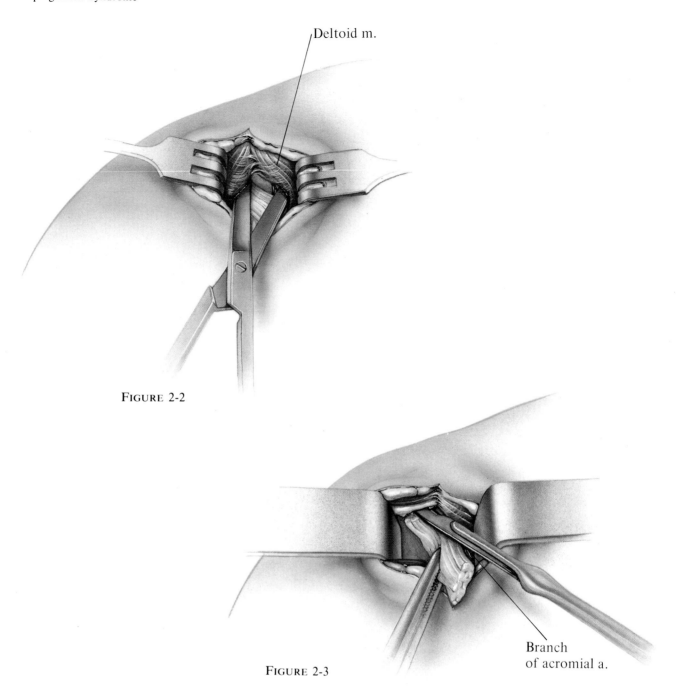

Deltoid m.

FIGURE 2-2

FIGURE 2-3

Branch
of acromial a.

Following irrigation, only the subcutaneous tissue and skin need be sutured. I prefer to use #2–0 Dexon interrupted sutures in the subcutaneous tissue and a subcuticular #4–0 clear Nylon suture in the skin. Next, apply Steri-strips in order to reinforce the suture and hold the wound edges together. Finally, apply adaptive dressing (4 × 4) and elastoplast dressing.

Postoperative Care and Rehabilitation

Postoperatively, allow the patient full use of the arm as soon as symptoms will allow. For the first day or two, a sling is frequently worn. But thereafter, the patient is encouraged to move the arm, particularly in patterns of internal and external rotation. After the first 3 days, encourage a full range of motion. One week following surgery, remove the skin sutures. Also start Codman's exercises. Three weeks after surgery the patient is usually capable of undertaking all athletic activities, but make certain that the return to activity is gradual (see Chap. 11).

Frequently, there is a considerable amount of muscle atrophy around the shoulder due to the lack of activity. In such cases, institute a good progressive resistance exercise, one that brings into play all of the muscles of the shoulder girdle. Continue progressive resistance exercises three times a week until there is a complete return of function.

Rotator Cuff Repair

General Considerations

Athletic activities that involve repetitive use of the arm above the horizontal level may produce an overuse syndrome. Neer has demonstrated that impingement of the vulnerable avascular region of the supraspinatus and biceps tendons occurs against the anterior edge of the acromion and the coracoacromial ligament.[3,4] The stages of this syndrome have been defined by several authors.[5,6] With repeated use the impingement can continue to actual tendon degeneration and rupture of the biceps and rotator cuff. In the early stages the diagnosis depends on a positive "impingement sign,"[3,4] and tenderness over either the biceps or the supraspinatus tendon. Both lesions are associated with a painful arc of abduction whenever the greater tuberosity is forward flexed against the anteroinferior edge of the acromion. Internal rotation of the humerus in this position causes impingement against the coracoacromial ligament. The surgical repair for the rotator cuff and the proximal biceps tendon will be described in sequence.

Surgical Procedure and Techniques

With the patient lying supine and a folded sheet placed into the median border of the scapula, prep the skin and drape the arm free.

Begin the skin incision at the posterior angle of the acromion process and carry it anteriorly across the top of the shoulder between the lateral edge of the acromion process and the acromioclavicular joint (Fig. 2-4). Next, carry this incision distally from the acromion, both laterally and medially, to give wide exposure to the underlying structures. Then carry the incision down to the fascia of the deltoid muscle and to the periosteum overlying the acromion process.

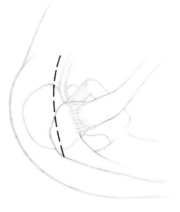

FIGURE 2-4

11

Deltoid m.

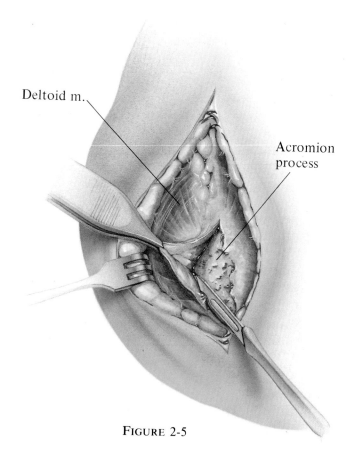

Acromion
process

FIGURE 2-5

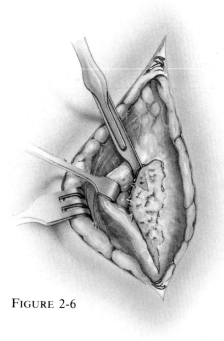

FIGURE 2-6

Begin the deep part of the incision at the posterolateral corner of the acromion process and incise down to bone to the anterior border of the acromion process. Either a scalpel blade or electrocautery knife may be used for this exposure. Take care, however, to be certain that the deep incision is over the acromion process and not laterally over the insertion of the deltoid muscle on the acromion. The reason for this is to develop a tough periosteal border for later reattachment of the deltoid to the acromion.

Once the incision is carried to the periosteum, elevate it laterally to the anterior and lateral borders of the acromion process by dissecting sharply with a #15 scalepl blade (Fig. 2-5). In this area, the periosteum is too adherent for the use of a periosteal elevator.

Once the periosteum is elevated to the lateral border of the acromion process and not beyond, continue the anterior aspect of the deep incision over the anterior border of the acromion process for approximately 5 mm and deep enough to allow access to the undersurface of the acromion, release the deltoid tendon fibers that insert underneath the acromion at the tendon bone junction. This will preserve the maximum amount of tendon tissues for later reapproximation of the deltoid to the acromion (Fig. 2-6). Because tendinous portion of the deltoid muscle in some individuals is not more than a few millimeters in thickness, try to be especially meticulous during this portion of the approach.

Once the deltoid is released in a semicircle from the acromion process, use scissors or an electrocautery knife to make an incision through the deltoid along one of the anterior raphe (Fig. 2-7). The deltoid muscle can then be retracted medially and laterally to expose the rotator cuff and the undersurface

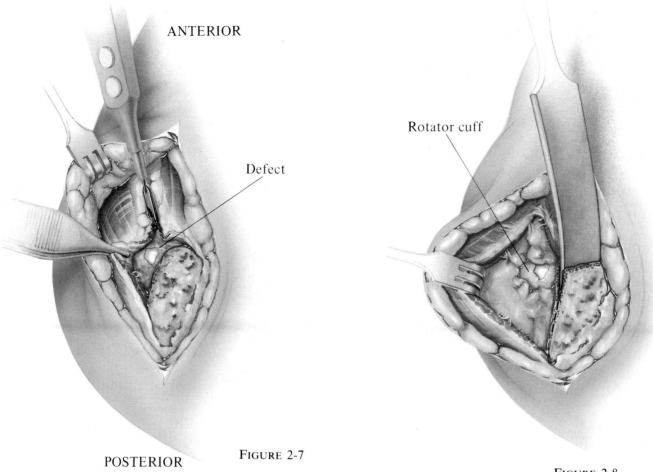

ANTERIOR

Defect

Rotator cuff

POSTERIOR   FIGURE 2-7

FIGURE 2-8

of the acromion process. Excise the subacromial bursa to expose the defect in the rotator cuff. If it is not seen immediately, rotate the humerus internally or externally to bring the tear into view. Prepare the acromion process for osteotomizing its anterior and inferior edge with a bone rongeur. Use the rongeur only to flatten the anterior and lateral edge. This will facilitate the positioning of the osteotome for the partial acromionectomy (Fig. 2-8). This cut is thicker anteriorly and tapers posteriorly.

Once the wedge of bone is removed from the undersurface of the acromion, the exposure to the rotator cuff is better. Excise the edges of the torn rotator cuff along their borders in order to have a fresh bleeding surface for repair. Prior to closure of the rotator cuff rent, retract the rotator cuff and examine the biceps tendon for any partial tears or evidence of synovitis around the bicipital groove.

Once the rotator cuff edges are prepared for closure, irrigate the wound routinely with Garamycin. Use #1 Ethibond suture for closure of the rotator cuff. The stitch can be either a simple through-and-through, a mattress, or a figure-of-eight (Fig. 2-9).

Occasionally, the tear leaves sufficient rotator still attached to the greater tuberosity and the closure can be accomplished with tendon-to-tendon sutures only. More commonly, the cuff is avulsed from the greater tuberosity and drill holes must be placed through it in order to reapproximate the rotator cuff. Frequently, the rotator cuff cannot be reapproximated without bringing the arm into abduction. If this is the case, splint the arm in abduction postoperatively.

13

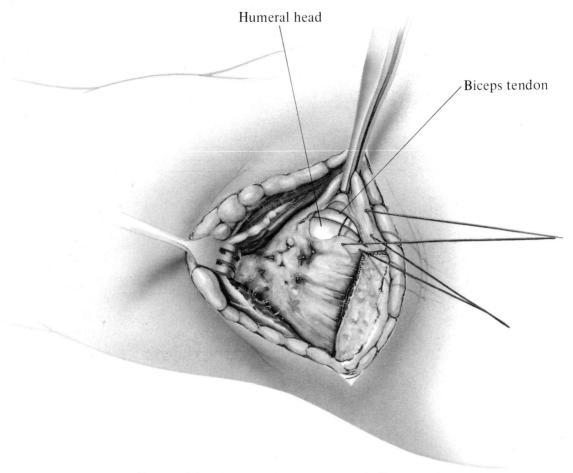

Humeral head

Biceps tendon

FIGURE 2-9.   Arm may be abducted to facilitate repair.

In cases where the tear is very large or of longstanding duration i.e., the "bald eagle" type, the rotator cuff tissues are contracted so that they cannot be reapproximated. Split the deltoid muscle a little further to mobilize the upper portion of the subscapularis muscle and tendon, to bring it cephalically to close the gap (Fig. 2-10). Sometimes the V-shaped defect in the subscapularis muscle can be partially or completely closed with interrupted sutures.

If, however, the rotator cuff defect is quite large and the contracted tissues cannot be freed up or are too inelastic to allow any reapproximation, fashion a GoreTex soft tissue patch and suture it into position. Pass a noncutting needle with a nonabsorbent suture through the graft and through the defect in the rotator cuff by using multiple interrupted sutures (Fig. 2-11). This graft should allow fibrous ingrowth into its substance and provide adequate coverage of previously exposed humeral head. However, since the rotator cuff muscle length is shortened, the repair may not result in an increase in strength.

Once the rotator cuff defect is closed, accomplish the very important reapproximation of the deltoid muscle by using #1 Ethibond sutures on a cutting needle and passing them through the acromion process (Fig. 2-12). Ideally, each stitch should exit along the flattened surface fashioned with the rongeur and then pass inferiorly through the substance of the deltoid tendon. The periosteal flap thereby pulls the deltoid more to the superior surface of the acromion process and not to the undersurface, which would thereby create a possible cause for further soft-tissue impingement against the underlying rotator cuff. Use multiple interrupted sutures to fashion a secure reapproxima-

Supraspinatus m.

Subscapularis m.

Cuff defect

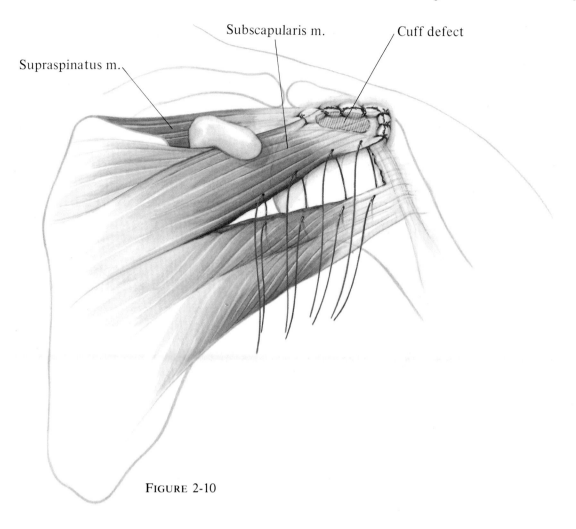

FIGURE 2-10

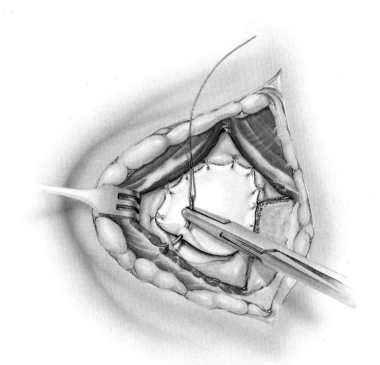

FIGURE 2-11. Arm abducted.

15

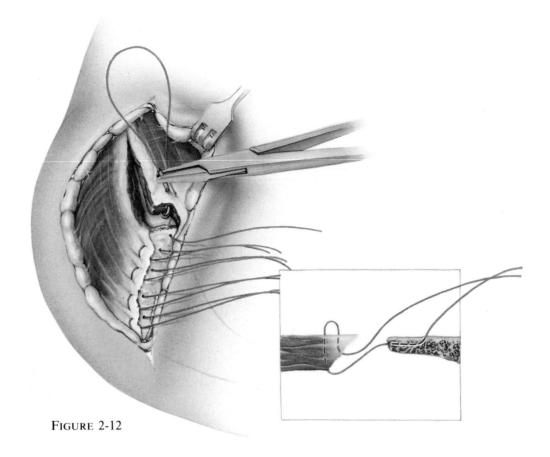

FIGURE 2-12

tion of the deltoid to the acromion process. Close the subcutaneous tissue in a routine fashion using #000 absorbable suture, close the skin with a running subcuticular clear nylon suture.

Postoperative Care and Rehabilitation

Place the patient in a shoulder immobilizer with the arm against the chest wall unless the repair of the defect requires a position of abduction. In that case, a type of airplane splint or pillow is used to decrease tension on the rotator cuff repair. At 12 days, remove the sutures and instruct the patient in passive abduction exercises. These should be performed daily at home or in therapy. Maintain immobilization from 4 to 6 weeks depending upon the size of the defect in the rotator cuff. Follow the rehabilitation program for the rotator cuff as described in Chapter 11 on rehabilitating the upper extremity.

Bicipital Tenodesis

General Considerations

If an attenuated or ruptured biceps tendon is encountered in the course of exploring the rotator cuff or of repairing the cuff, a tenodesis of the biceps can be accomplished through the same incision. In the older athlete, a rupture

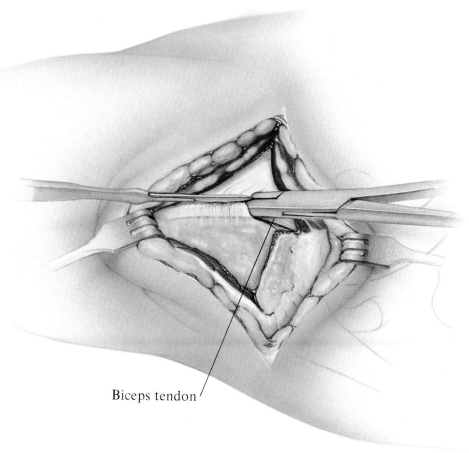

Biceps tendon

FIGURE 2-13

of the long head of the biceps is related to impingment; however, in the younger competitor, the tendon tears with a violent episode of trauma.[6,7]

Surgical Procedure and Techniques

This procedure sometimes requires some further splitting of the deltoid. Here care must be taken not to approach the axillary nerve too closely. By rotating the humerus, the biceps groove can be directly palpated and visualized. And by flexing the elbow and compressing the biceps muscle from distal to proximal, the ruptured portion of the biceps tendon can usually either be visualized or grasped with an instrument. If neither of these steps can be achieved, open the covering over the biceps groove by sharp incision (Fig. 2-13). If the tendon has ruptured, then remove the remaining portion of the biceps tendon from the joint through a split in the rotator cuff.

If the tendon is greatly attenuated but intact, remove it from its origin along the glenoid through a split in the rotator cuff at the junction of the supraspinatus and the subscapularis muscles (Fig. 2-14). The length of tendon available will determine the site of the drill holes in the bicipital groove. If the tendon is of sufficient length, place them proximally; if it is ruptured and there is only a short portion available, place them more distally. Be sure to place the two drill holes 1.5 cm apart and curette them to facilitate the passing of the biceps tendon from distal to proximal (Fig. 2-15).

Fold the tendon distally and suture it with #1 Ethibond. Be sure to suture the back of the tendon on itself and its sides to the cut edges of the tissue of the bicipital groove (Fig. 2-16).

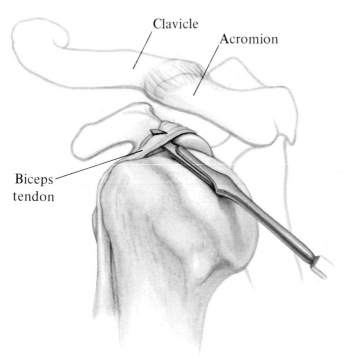

Clavicle

Acromion

Biceps
tendon

FIGURE 2-14.   Lateral view.

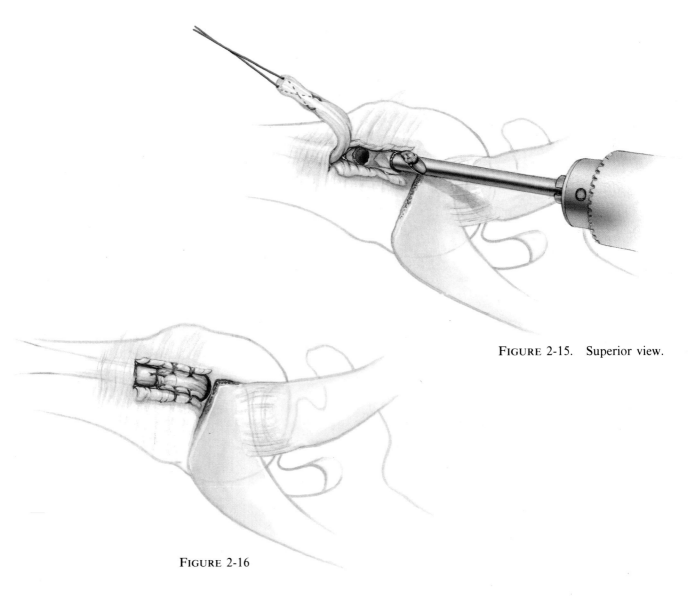

FIGURE 2-15.   Superior view.

FIGURE 2-16

References

Coracoacromial Ligament Resection

1. Jackson DW: Chronic rotator cuff impingement in the throwing athlete. *Am J Sports Med* 1976;4:231–240.
2. Strizak AM, Dawzig L, et al: Staple T: Subacromial bursography: An anatomic and clinical study. Presented at American Orthopaedic Society for Sports Medicine, Las Vegas, NV, February 1980.
3. Hawkins RJ, Kennedy JC: Impingement syndrome in athletes. *Am J Sports Med* 1980;8:151–158.

Rotator Cuff Repair

4. Neer CS: Anterior acromioplasty for chronic impingement syndrome in the shoulder. *J Bone Jt Surg* 1972;54A:41–50.
5. Jobe FW: Serious rotator calf injuries. *Clin Sports Med* 1983;2:407.

Bicipital Tenodesis

6. Penny JN, Welsh RP: Shoulder impingement syndromes in athletes and their surgical management. *Am J Sports Med* 1981;9:11–15.
7. Del Pizzo W, Norwood LA, et al: Rupture of the biceps tendon in gymnastics: a case report. *Am J Sports Med* 1978;6:283–286.

Additional Reading

Coracoacromial Ligament Resection

Dominguez RH: Coracoacromial ligament resection for severe swimmer's shoulder, in Eridsson B, Furberg B (eds): *Swimming Medicine* IV Baltimore, University Park Press, 1978, pp. 110–114.
Johansson JE, Barringtoon TW: Coracoacromial ligament division. *Am J Sports Med* 1984;12:138–141.

Rotator Cuff

Bassett RW, Cofield RH: Acute tears of the rotator cuff. The timing of surgical repair. *Clin Orthop* 1983;175:18–24.
De Orio JK, Cofield RH: Results of a second attempt at surgical repair of a failed initial rotator cuff repair. *J Bone Jt Surg* 1984;66A:563–567.
Jobe FW, Moynes DR: Delineation of diagnostic criteria and a rehabilitation program for rotator cuff injuries. *Am J Sports Med* 1982;10:336–339.
Neer CS, Craig EV, Fukuda H: Cuff tear arthropathy. *J Bone JT Surg* 1983;65A:1232–1244.
Post M, Silver R, Singh M: Rotator cuff tear-diagnosis and treatment. *Clin Orthop* 1983;173:78–91.

Bicipital Tenodesis

Dines D, Warren RF, Inglis AE: Surgical treatment of lesions of the long head of the biceps. *Clin Orthop* 1982;164:165–171.
Haeri GB, Wiley AM: Shoulder impingement syndrome: Results of operative release. *Clin Orthop* 1982;168:128–132.
O'Donoghue DH: Subluxing biceps tendon in the athlete. *Clin Orthop* 1982;164:26–29.

3 Anterior Reconstruction

Stephen J. Lombardo

Modified Bristow Procedure

General Considerations

The Bristow procedure, in which the distal portion of the coracoid process is sutured to the anterior aspect of the scapular neck through a transversely sectioned subscapularis muscle, was described in 1958[3] for anterior instability of the shoulder. Mead[5] modified that procedure by affixing the bone block to the anterior glenoid rim with a screw. In recent years, this modified Bristow procedure has gained in popularity. Since 1971, over 500 procedures have been performed in our office for recurrent anterior shoulder subluxation/dislocation. The procedure has proved to be effective with an approximate recurrence rate of 2 to 3 percent.[1,2,4] It has not, however, permitted athletes who are engaged in sports that feature throwing as an activity to return to their preinjury functional level. Other procedures used in this select group of athletes have likewise been unrewarding to date.

Surgical Procedure and Techniques

Place the patient in a supine position with a small pillow or one-half surgical sheet beneath the involved scapula. The axilla of the patient is at the side of the operating table. Abduct the extremity from 40 to 50 degrees and place on an armboard. The extremity should be at the midpoint of the board. This will prevent unnecessary backstrain on the surgeon or assistant. The anesthesiologist's equipment should be to the uninvolved side of the patient. It is usually necessary to have the patient entubated. Drape the involved extremity free to permit movement of the extremity during the procedure. Stand at the axillary side of the patient and have your assistant stand on the acromial side. A second assistant or nurse may stand on the opposite side of the table.

Start the deltopectoral incision approximately from 2 to 3 cm distal and lateral to the palpable coracoid process and extend it approximately 8 cm to the axilla (Fig. 3-1). Forward flexion and adduction of the extremity will facilitate palpation of the less prominent coracoid process. In women, the axillary incision can be used for cosmesis. This incision is deltopectoral in

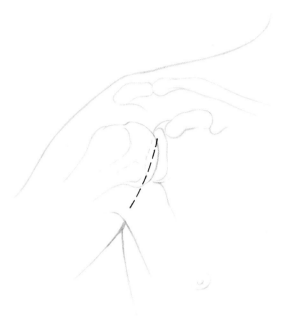

nature but more distal and directed into the axilla so that the incision is not visible when the arm is at the side. Following the skin incision, undermine the subcutaneous tissues. In doing so, visualize the deltopectoral groove by studying the orientation of the fibers of the deltoid and the pectoralis major muscle. A small amount of adipose tissue is usually present in the interval. (If you have difficulty in identifying this interval, direct the dissection more distally.) Within this interval, the cephalic vein can be identified and refected laterally with the deltoid muscle.

If the vein cannot be identified, the tissue plane in the area of the deltopectoral region should be developed and carried down to the fascia overlying the conjoined tendon and coracoid process. Do this part of the procedure with firm gentle pressure with the index finger placed medially and then laterally and brought superior to the coracoid and inferior to the fascia of the pectoralis major muscle over the proximal humerus.

If firm fibrous bands are encountered deep to the muscles, it is necessary to dissect them sharply to gain mobility of these tissues. It is important to undermine the deltoid and pectoral muscles both bluntly and sharply. This permits easier retraction. Richardson's or Goulet retractors can be used to reflect the deltoid muscle laterally and the pectoralis major muscle medially. In the case of muscular athletes, Richardson's are preferable since more tissue can be retracted with its longer and wider blade.

Once the deltoid and pectoralis are reflected, the conjoined tendon and coracoid can then be visualized. Use sharp dissection to excise a sufficient amount of soft tissue along the medial and lateral portion of the conjoined tendon. This maneuver is necessary both to allow reflection of the coracoid process and conjoined tendon as one unit distally and to permit adequate visualization of the underlying subscapularis muscle. This dissection can be performed sharply with the use of a long handled #15 blade or dissecting scissors. Usually 6 to 8 cm of dissection is necessary along the borders of the conjoined tendon. At the coracoid process, free the soft tissue attachment medially and laterally for 1.5 to 2 cm along the pectoralis minor muscle attachment on the medial side and the coracoacromial ligament laterally. Then, with blunt and/or sharp dissection, incise the fascia overlying the supe-

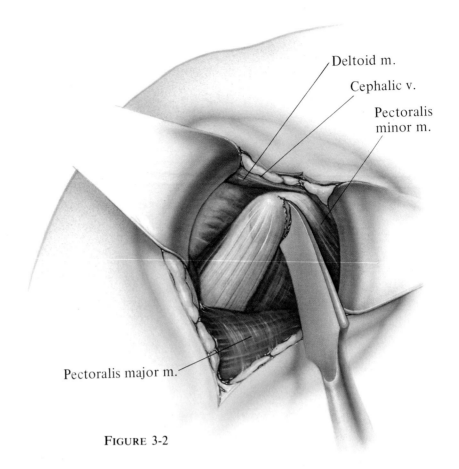

Deltoid m.

Cephalic v.

Pectoralis
minor m.

Pectoralis major m.

FIGURE 3-2

rior part of the coracoid process for 1 to 1.5 cm from the tip. This helps to delineate the area of the coracoid process that will be osteotomized and reflected with the attached conjoined tendon.

To osteotomize the coracoid processes, use a ½- or ¾-inch curved osteotome (Fig. 3-2). It is necessary to place the osteotome deep to the conjoined tendon in a position so that a 1 to 1.5 cm length of the coracoid can be osteotomized. A little smaller length is acceptable. As long as the bone block accepts the screw, the length is sufficient.

I prefer to place the osteotome from an inferior to superior direction on the coracoid process. Usually I am able to achieve this placement by directing the osteotome from an inferior medial direction to superior lateral direction. In the case of men with heavily muscled chest walls or women with large breasts, it may be better to use an inferior lateral to superior medial direction. In every case, a critical aspect of this step is proper placement of the osteotome.

Once the mallet is utilized and the osteotomy is begun, it should be continued to completion. A major pitfall is to remove the osteotome *before* the cut is completed. Difficulty can then be encountered in trying to replace the osteotome. Because young athletic individuals have very hard bone, use a 3 pound mallet. Be sure to palpate the osteotome and its relationship to the coracoid process so that the breadth of the osteotome will cut through the entire width of the coracoid. Once the osteotomy is complete, soft tissues may remain attached to the coracoid process. After gently grabbing the conjoined tendon at its attachment to the coracoid with Kocher's clamps, make a sharp dissection of these attachments. Once this is achieved, reflect the coracoid and conjoined tendon distally in order to visualize the underlying subscapularis tendon and muscle. At this point, remove any bony spikes on the detached or remaining coracoid with rongeurs.

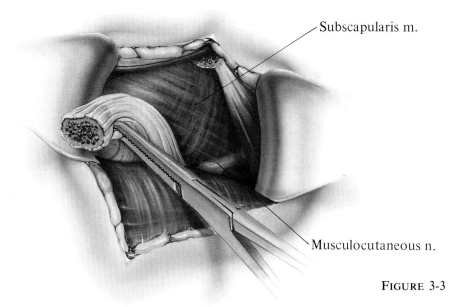

Subscapularis m.

Musculocutaneous n.

FIGURE 3-3

The musculocutaneous nerve inserts on the conjoined tendon at a varied distance of 2 to 7 cm from the coracoid process. Be careful not to place undue traction on the coracoid process (Fig. 3-3). Once the coracoid process and conjoined tendon are reflected distally, place them within the depth of the wound and reflect them from the operative field with a 4 × 4 sponge. (Inform the nurse that a sponge is present in the wound.) Now, identify the subscapularis muscle and split it in line with its fibers from lateral to medial. The level of the split is approximately the middle half to lower one-third, and the venous plexus marks the lower border of the subscapularis muscle.

An important landmark for splitting the subscapularis muscle is the anterior face of the glenoid. This is usually best identified by taking the extremity and flexing it forward. This maneuver places the humeral head in the posterior direction and prevents it from obstructing the palpating of the anterior face of the glenoid. The common tendency during this phase of the procedure—and one that should be avoided—is to start the dissection laterally and to let the knife drift inferior medial rather than to keep it in a straight medial direction. Repeated palpation of the anterior face of the glenoid will eliminate this error. The lateral aspect of this phase of the dissection should be achieved without any difficulty. The only area of concern is the biceps tendon, and this can be readily palpated with internal rotation of the humerus. If the arm is held in a 20 to 30 degrees of abduction, and rotated externally, the tendon will be removed from the operative field.

The sequence of the procedure involving the subscapularis muscle is:

1. Dissect the overlying fascia of the subscapularis muscle sharply. Doing this with a "hot knife" will prevent bleeding.
2. Once the muscle of the subscapularis muscle is exposed, use a ¾-inch periosteal elevator to reflect it from the overlying capsule in a superior and inferior direction.
3. After grasping the capsule with a Kocher's clamp, perform an arthrotomy with sharp dissection (Fig. 3-4).

Carry the dissection from lateral to medial down to the anterior face of the glenoid, where a Bankart lesion is usually present. When entering through the capsule, be careful; otherwise, the articular surface of the humeral head can be scored.

23

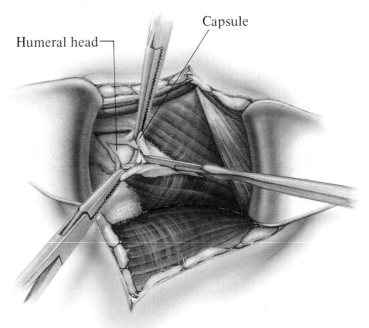

Humeral head

Capsule

FIGURE 3-4

Next, incise the labrum and capsule along the anterior face of the glenoid and reflect them in a superior medial and an inferior medial direction. Do this with sharp dissection for a distance of 2 to 3 cm on the anterior face of the glenoid. Sometimes an avulsion fracture is present on the anterior face of the glenoid. In these cases, reflect the fracture with the capsule and labrum so that the remaining intact anterior glenoid face can be prepared for placement of the coracoid bone block. (In over 500 cases, we have had no problems with an insufficient amount of articular surface and bone remaining on the glenoid.) By keeping the dissection deep to the subscapularis muscle, you will avoid the medial neurovascular bundle and thus, not damage it.

Once the glenoid has been prepared, insert a right-angled humeral-head retractor between the glenoid and the humeral head. Now, in order to retract the humeral head posteriorly and laterally to give an excellent view of the articular surface of the glenoid, place the humeral-head retractor so that is distracts and depresses the humeral head by axial traction on the extremity at 30 degrees of abduction. The curve of the retractor, which contours to the humeral head, facilitates its placement as does gentle traction and internal rotation of the humeral head while the retractor is inserted. Reflect the superior and inferior leaves of the glenoid labrum and capsule with attached clamps. Next, place a "devil's pitchfork" (three-pronged retractor) on the anterior face of the glenoid, but take care not to do this blindly; otherwise, neurovascular damage may result since medial to dissection is the brachial plexus and vascular bundle. If there is any concern about placement of a three-pronged retractor during the procedure, use a large periosteal elevator for retraction by placing it along the bony surface of the anterior glenoid. It is also possible to use an upright retractor, which does not have the prongs of the devil's pitchfork.

Now, utilize a 3.2-mm drill point to make a hole in an anterior posterior direction on the glenoid approximately 2 cm away from the articular surface of the glenoid (Fig. 3-5). Align the direction of the drill hole parallel to the face of the glenoid. This is easily achieved by depressing the humeral head with the retractor in place and visualizing the plane of the articular surface of the glenoid. Take care that the drill hole does not bind against the devil's

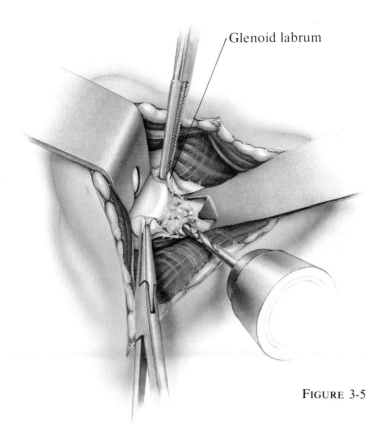

Glenoid labrum

FIGURE 3-5

pitchfork; otherwise, metal shavings can be fragmented from contact between the two instruments. While the drill hole is being made from the anterior to the posterior direction, it is also important to avoid putting a great deal of manual pressure on the drill; otherwise, the drill may piston through the posterior cortex of the glenoid. To be sure that the drill hole goes through the entire depth of the scapular neck, use a depth gauge to measure the length of the hole.

After the screw hole is completed in the glenoid, prepare the remaining face of the glenoid, which usually measures about 3 by 2 cm. Do this with either a small osteotome or a drill to create bleeding bone so that fixation of the bone block to the anterior face of the glenoid will be in a relatively vascular bed.

Next, remove the 4 × 4 sponge in the distal depth of the wound and then grasp the coracoid process that has been resected with the conjoined tendon and make a drill hole through it. (The assistant usually does this part of the procedure.) This step will eliminate undue traction on the coracoid process and conjoined tendon. As a result, a drill hole is more readily performed from the cut surface of the coracoid process to its tip. Once the same 3.2-mm drill penetrates the entire length of the coracoid process, use a knife to free the tissue around the drill point so that when the screw is placed, the hole is readily found. (On one occasion, because of a lack of adequate diameter of the bone block, it was necessary to fix the bone block to the anterior face of the glenoid by placing the drill hole from a medial to lateral direction through the coracoid process. In all other cases, the conventional way has been adequate.) The depth of the drill hole through the coracoid process usually measures 14 mm or less. The AO (*Arbeitsgemeinschaft für Osteosynthesefragen*) malleolar screw that is to be affixed has a combined length of the two drill holes and is usually between 30 and 45 mm overall.

Malleolar screws come in 5.0 mm increments. In the earlier part of our series of operations, we used the screw length closest to the combined measurement. This choice proved unsatisfactory because screws that protrude through the posterior cortex of the glenoid create a bursa and discomfort in some patients. I thus now use the lesser screw length to the measured distance. For example, if the combined measurement is 39 mm, then a 35 mm screw is utilized. In these cases, I feel the posterior cortex is still penetrated, since the head and neck of the screw countersinks within the coracoid process from 3 to 4 mm. In no cases have I had further problems with posterior shoulder discomfort; nor has the lesser screw length been so inadequate that it results in screw migration.

Once a screw of the proper length is selected, inspect the joint and do a manual palpation for loose fragments and labral lesions. Finally, irrigate the joint profusely with antibiotic solution.

Now, hold the coracoid process by its tendinous part with a Kocher's clamp. Be careful not to gasp the bone block with the Kocher's or any other instrument; for, on a number of occasions when this has been done, the bone block has fractured. In these cases, it is then necessary to staple the bone block or to suture it to the anterior face of the glenoid.

The smooth part of the malleolar screw should engage the coracoid process to achieve a lag effect. Place the screw through the coracoid process and the anterior face of the glenoid (Fig. 3-6). It is very important that the instruments reflecting the tissue on the anterior face of the glenoid do not obstruct or impinge upon the bone block as it is fixed. This, too, can create a fracture of the coracoid process.

Once the screw is in place and the bone block is fixed, be sure that there is no overhang of the bone block. If there is overhang and the bone block is longer in one plane than another, loosen the screw and rotate the bone block so that the narrowest portion of the bone block is in a medial lateral direction. This usually permits satisfactory bone contact without overhang.

If the reflected glenoid labrum and tissue are unduly loose and have the potential of impingement within the joint, then suture the labrum and tissue to the tendinous portion of the conjoined tendon. This can be achieved with a #00 or #0 absorbable suture. Once again, irrigate the wound profusely with Garamycin solution. With two absorbable sutures, reapproximate the fascia overlying the subscapularis muscle. This is done for hemostasis. Next, place a sponge deep to the deltopectoral muscles and remove the instruments. Then, remove the sponge, identify any bleeding, and stop it with the use of a Bovie (electrocautery knife). Gelfoam is not ordinarily used.

Do the closure of the fascia overlying the deltopectoral and subcutaneous tissue with #000 absorable sutures and the skin with the running #0000 subcuticular nylon suture and Steri-strips applied to the skin.

It is important to pad the axilla with ABD pads to prevent skin maceration. Place 4 × 8-inch sponges over the incision followed by elastic tape and reinforce with 2-inch tape on the edges. Place the extremity in a sling. Before removing the patient from the operating room, confirm the sponge and needle count twice.

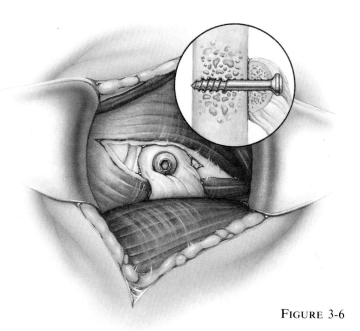

FIGURE 3-6

Postoperative Care and Rehabilitation

The postoperative management includes elbow motion on Day 1 and gentle pendulum exercise on Day 2. Physical therapy for a range of active motion and strengthening exercises starts at 3 weeks. Contact and throwing activities are not allowed for 4 to 6 months (Chap. 11).

Anterior Staple Capsulorrhaphy

General Considerations

An alternative to the modified Bristow procedure for correcting recurrent subluxation and dislocations of the shoulder in throwing athletes is anterior staple capsulorrhaphy. The early results of this alternative procedure do not show that athletes return to their preinjury level of function.

Surgical Procedure and Techniques

The procedure is done through either a deltopectoral or an axillary approach. Incise the conjoined tendon transversely 2 to 3 cm from the coracoid process and reflect it distally (Fig. 3-7). Next, split the subscapularis muscle down to the anterior capsule longitudinally from lateral to medial to the edge of the anterior glenoid rim and reflect the muscle both superiorly and inferiorly with a periosteal elevator (Fig. 3-8).

Now, incise the capsule longitudinally from lateral to medial before inspecting and probing the incision with a nerve hook for Bankart, Hill-Sachs, or labral lesions (Fig. 3-9). When a Bankart lesion is present, curette the anterior glenoid deep to the anterior capsule. Fix the anterior capsule to the glenoid with a double-pronged serrated staple. Placement of the staple is approximately 1 cm medial to the glenohumeral joint (Fig. 3-10). Reapproximate the fascia overlying the subscapularis muscle and the conjoined tendon with figure-of-eight absorbable sutures (Fig. 3-11). Close the deltopectoral fascia and subcuta-

27

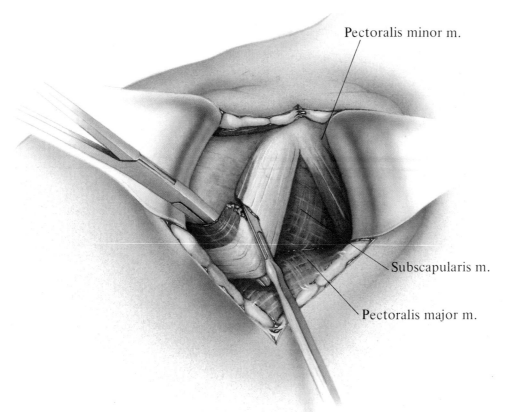

Pectoralis minor m.

Subscapularis m.

Pectoralis major m.

FIGURE 3-7

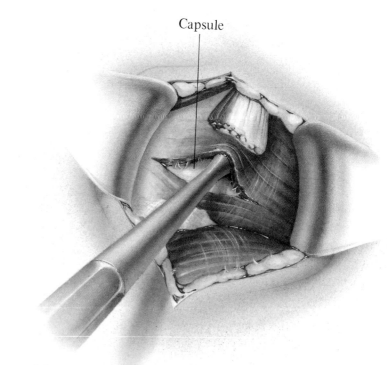

Capsule

FIGURE 3-8

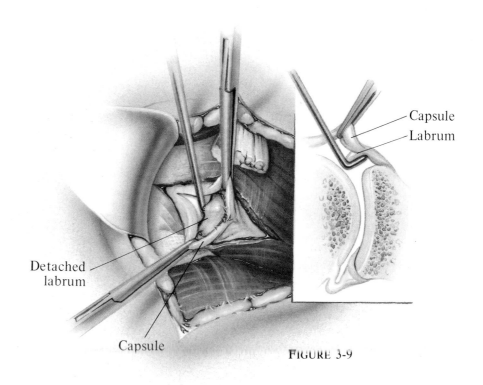

Capsule

Labrum

Detached
labrum

Capsule

FIGURE 3-9

Edge of glenoid

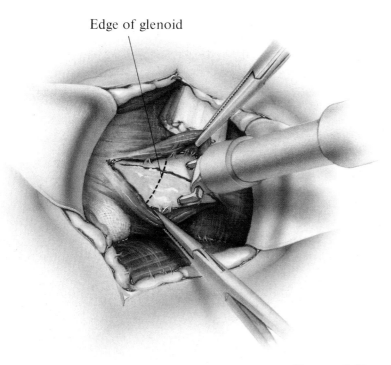

FIGURE 3-10

29

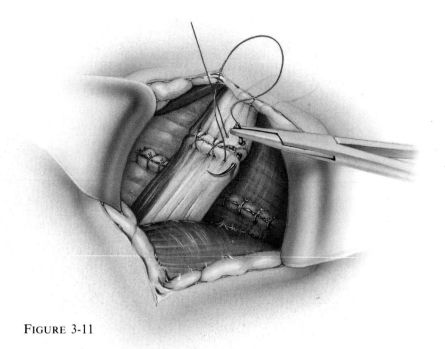

FIGURE 3-11

neous tissue with absorbable sutures. To complete the procedure, close the skin with #4–0 nylon.

Use a sling postoperatively, initiate a graduated therapy program at 1 to 2 weeks. Have the patient resume full activities only after 4 to 6 months (Chap. 11).

References

1. Barry TP, Lombardo SJ, et al: The coracoid transfer for recurrent anterior instability of the shoulder in adolescents. *J Bone Jt Surg* 1985;67A:383–387.
2. Collins HR, Wilde AH: Shoulder instability in athletics. *Orthop Clin North Am,* 1973;4:3:759–774.
3. Helfet, AJ: Coracoid transplantation for recurring dislocation of the shoulder. *J Bone Jt Surg,* 1958;40B:198–202.
4. Lombardo, SJ, Kerlan RK, et al: The modified Bristow procedure for recurrent dislocation of the shoulder. *J Bone Joint Surg* 1976,58A:256 261.
5. Sweeney, HJ, Mead NC, et: Fourteen Year's Experience with the modified Bristow Procedure for Recurrent Anterior dislocation of the shoulder, Read at the annual meeting of the American Academy of Orthopedic Surgery San Francisco Calif, Mar 5, 1975.

Additional Reading

Chen SK, Perry J, et al: Elbow flexion analysis in Bristow patients. A preliminary report. *Am J Sports Med* 1984;12:347–350.
Hill JA, Lombardo SJ, et al: The modified Bristow-Helfet procedure for recurrent anterior shoulder subluxations and dislocations. *Am J Sports Med* 1981;9:283–287.
Mizuno K, Hirohata K· Diagnosis of recurrent traumatic anterior subluxation of the shoulder. *Clin Orthop* 1983;179:160–167.
Pappas AM, Goss TP, Kleinman PK. Symptomatic shoulder instability due to lesions of the glenoid labrum. *Am J Sports Med* 1983;11:279–288.
Rowe CR, Zarins B, Cuillo JV: Recurrent anterior dislocation of the shoulder after surgical repair. *J Bone Jt Surg* 1984;66A:159–168.

Warren RF: Subluxation of the shoulder in athletes. *Clin Sports Med* 1983;2:339–354.

Zarins B, Rowe CR: Current concepts in the diagnosis and treatment of shoulder instability in athletes. *Med Sci Sports Exerc* 1984;16(5):444–448.

Zuckerman JD, Matsen FA: Complications about the glenohumeral joint related to the use of screws and staples. *J Bone Jt Surg* 1984;66A:175–180.

4 Posterior Reconstruction

James E. Tibone

General Considerations

To the orthopedist, the approach to the posterior shoulder area is not so familiar as that to the anterior shoulder.[1-3] In the field of sports medicine, however, it is necessary to be able to expose the posterior aspect of the shoulder atraumatically in order to treat recurrent posterior subluxations/dislocations of the shoulder and to debride calcium and bone spurs in this area. The diagnosis of posterior shoulder instability is usually difficult, but it can be made with repeated examination of the athlete.[4,5]

The athlete will usually complain of pain in the posterior aspect of his shoulder or of his arm "going dead." Usually, he will demonstrate this as occurring in the follow-through stage of the throwing motion. On physical examination, the instability can commonly be demonstrated by forward flexing and by internally rotating and adducting the arm.[5] An axillary lateral radiograph taken in this position may also demonstrate the posterior instability. It is important to compare the involved shoulder with the contralateral arm because some athletes have ligamentous laxity. The indication for a posterior shoulder stabilization is an athlete who does not respond to at least 6 months of conservative care, including anti-inflammatory medicines, rest, and muscle strengthening involving the posterior rotator cuff area. The instability, in itself, is not an indication for surgery, but the presence of persistent pain is.[4,5] A staple capsulorrhaphy is usually done to repair the posterior shoulder instability. This procedure is contraindicated in athletes who have ligamentous laxity since there is a high rate of failure in these individuals. The staple capsulorrhaphy is usually successful in preventing recurrent subluxation/dislocation, but it is unpredictable in allowing an athlete to return to his former throwing status.[5]

Surgical Procedure and Techniques

Place the patient on the operating table in the lateral decubitus position with the involved shoulder superior; hold him in position with an inflatable Olympic Vac-Pac Surgical Positioning System "bean bag" and kidney rest. Place the operating table itself on a slightly reversed Trendelenburg position.

Make a saber incision at the superior aspect of the shoulder. This incision starts at the acromioclavicular joint and extends posteriorly approximately

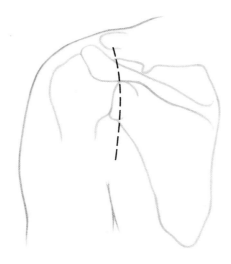

FIGURE 4-1

8 cm into the posterior axillary fold (Fig. 4-1). Undermine the subcutaneous tissues to expose the deltoid muscle attachment to the acromion and the spine of the scapula. Next, identify the fascial raphe between the middle and posterior third of the deltoid muscle and slit it distally and posteriorly up to 4 cm (Fig. 4-2). In doing so, take care to avoid the axillary nerve that enters the deltoid muscle at the inferior border of the teres minor muscle. Using sharp dissection, reflect the deltoid from the scapular spine and posterior aspect of the acromion. The deltoid attachment adheres to the infraspinatus

Deltoid raphe

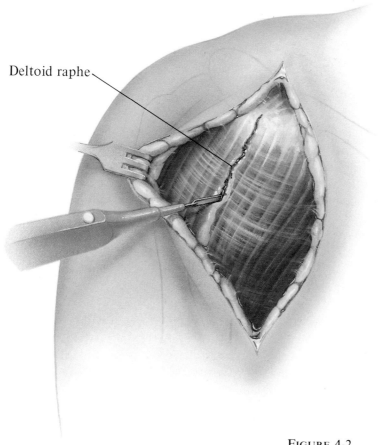

FIGURE 4-2

33

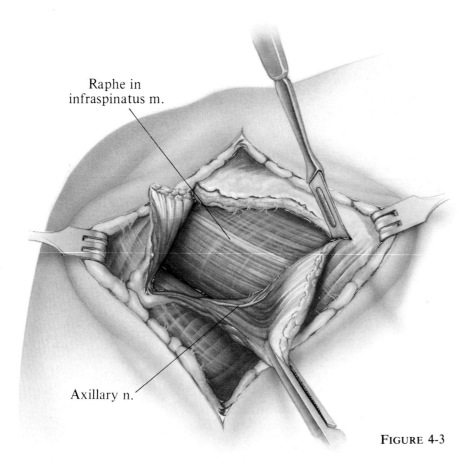

Raphe in
infraspinatus m.

Axillary n.

FIGURE 4-3

attachment to the spine of the scapula. Thus, it is easier to find the plane between these two muscles by starting out laterally in the area of the acromion with the sharp dissection (Fig. 4-3).

After the deltoid muscle is reflected, the teres minor and infraspinatus muscles are encountered below the fascia of the deltoid. The infraspinatus is a bipennate muscle with a raphe between its two heads. This raphe can be confused with the interval between the infraspinatus and teres minor muscles. The true interval between the infraspinatus and teres minor muscles is below this raphe, which is below the inferior head of the infraspinatus.

With blunt dissection in line with its fiber, develop the interval between the teres minor and infraspinatus muscles by exposing the posterior shoulder capsule (Fig. 4-4). Make an arthrotomy in the posterior capsule in the same direction as the fibers of the infraspinatus and teres minor muscles. This allows inspection of the joint.

At this point, debride bone spurs on the posterior glenoid. A posterior Bankart lesion is usually found with the labrum detached from the posterior glenoid. Strip the posterior capsule further off the posterior glenoid and the labrum. If the labrum is torn, remove it (Fig. 4-5).

Roughen the bone on the posterior glenoid labrum with curettes and rongeurs, and hold the two leaves of the posterior capsule with Kocher's clamps while positioning a barbed Richards' 1-inch staple. It is usually necessary to make drill holes through the cortex of the posterior glenoid with a $\frac{7}{64}$-inch drill bit to allow the staple to be positioned (Fig. 4-6). (The holes should be marked with a staple prior to drilling).

Place the staple approximately 1 cm from the glenoid rim and direct it slightly medially to avoid entering the joint. The reason for this approach

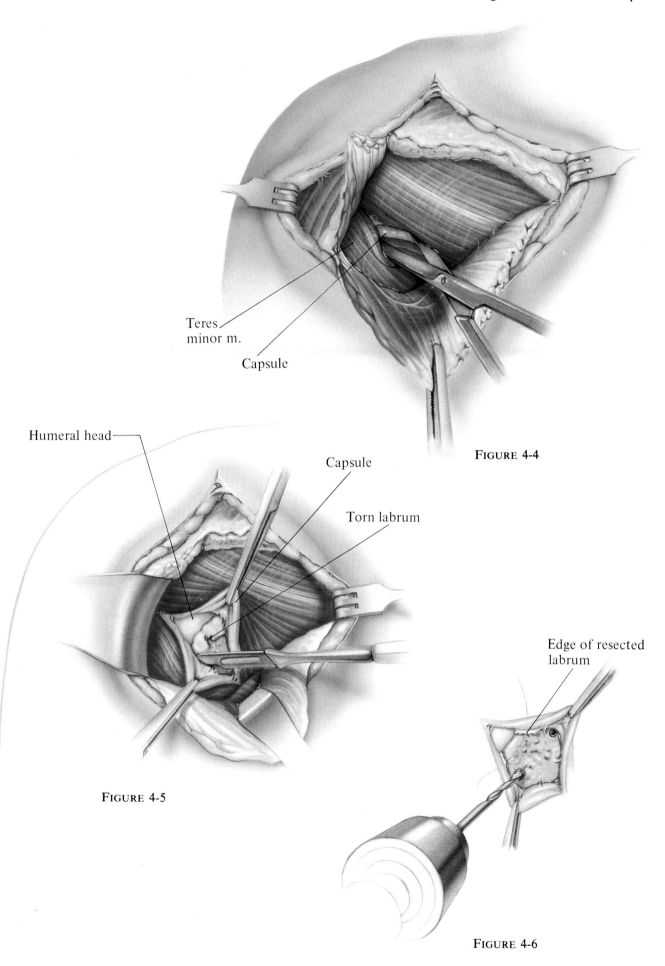

Teres
minor m.

Capsule

FIGURE 4-4

Humeral head

Capsule

Torn labrum

Edge of resected
labrum

FIGURE 4-5

FIGURE 4-6

Inferior capsule

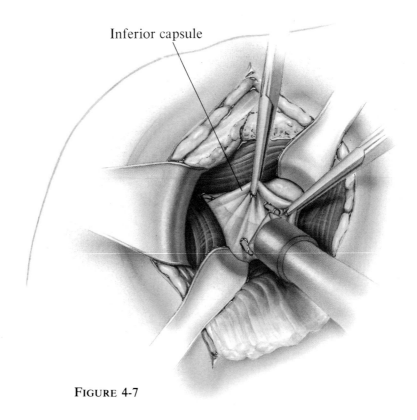

FIGURE 4-7

is the glenoid, which is usually anteverted in relationship to the sagittal plane of the body. Next, fix the posterior capsule to the posterior glenoid with the staple and close the capsule with horizontal mattress sutures by using #1 Vicryl suture (Fig. 4-7).

If there is inferior instability as well as posterior instability, develop the inferior capsule and advance it as far superiorly as possible to eliminate the inferior capsular pouch. No sutures are needed between the teres minor and infraspinatus muscles, and these muscles are not imbricated. Repair the deltoid muscle into the bone of the spine and the acromion with #1 Ethibond sutures on a small cutting needle (Fig. 4-8). Finally, close the skin and subcutaneous tissues in routine fashion and apply a compressive dressing.

Postoperative Care and Rehabilitation

Postoperatively, immobilize the patient in a sling for at least 3 weeks. In individuals who have lax ligaments and show inferior instability, increase the period of immobilization from 6 to 8 weeks. After this procedure, it is not necessary to immobilize the patient in external rotation.

Following the immobilization in the sling, start the patient on Codman's exercises and active and active assisted range of motion exercises. In another 4 weeks, begin the strengthening process with light weights of only 2 pounds to strengthen the posterior rotator cuff muscles of the infraspinatus and teres minor muscles as well as the posterior deltoid muscle. At 12 weeks following surgery, begin a program to strengthen the entire shoulder girdle (Chap. 11). For 6 months following the surgery, deny the patient all participation in sports.

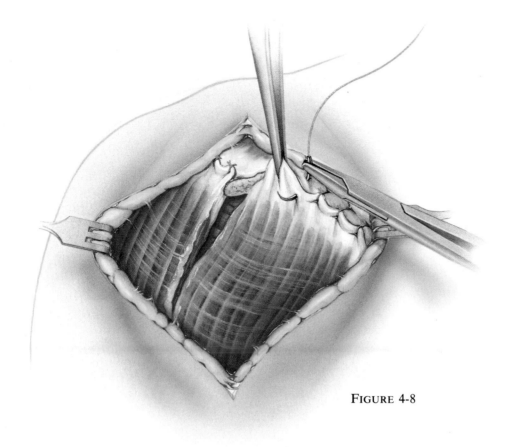

FIGURE 4-8

References

1. Rowe CR: Prognosis in dislocations of the shoulder. *J Bone Jt Surg* 1956;38A:957–977.
2. Dorgan JA: Posterior dislocation of the shoulder. *Am J Surg* 1955;58:890–900.
3. Roberts A, Wickstrom J: Prognosis of posterior dislocation of the shoulder. *Acta Orthop Scand* 1971;42:328–337.
4. Tibone JE, Prietto C, et al: Staple capsulorrhaphy for recurrent posterior shoulder dislocation. *Am J Sports Med* 1981;9:135–139.

Additional Reading

Hawkins RJ, Koppert G, Johnston G: Recurrent posterior instability (subluxation) of the shoulder. *J Bone Jt Surg* 1984;66A:169–174.

Neer CS, Foster CR: Inferior capsular shift for involuntary and multidirectional instability of the shoulder. A preliminary report. *J Bone Jt Surg* 1980;62A:897–908.

Elbow

II

5 Arthroscopy

Lewis A. Yocum

General Considerations

Like the knee, shoulder, and ankle, the elbow can be evaluated arthroscopically. Arthroscopy gives the surgeon the opportunity to assay thoroughly the articular surfaces of the joint. Loose bodies can be removed,[1] arthritis staged, and fractures assessed.[2] In addition, the procedure can be carried out under local, regional, or general anesthetic. However, a thorough understanding of the anatomy of the elbow, especially the radial nerve and its motor branch, is essential if arthroscopy is to prove fruitful.[3]

Surgical Procedure and Techniques

After effective anesthesia is instituted, check the elbow for range of motion and stress the ulnar collateral ligament. Prepare the arm in the usual fashion, draping it free. A pneumatic cuff is optional, but should be present whether

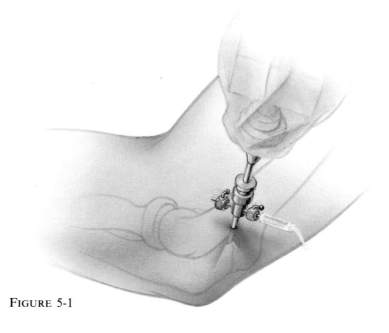

FIGURE 5-1

Radial n.

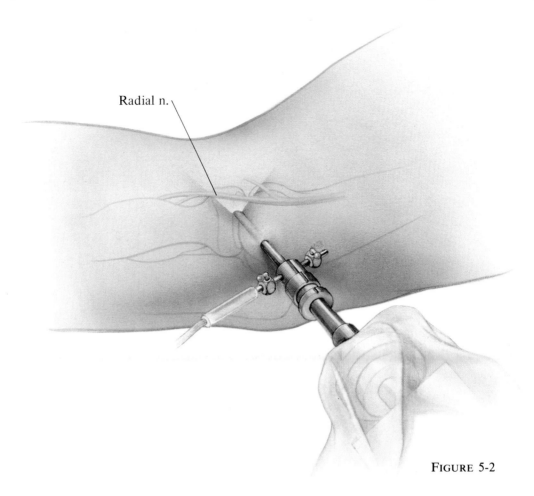

FIGURE 5-2

it is used or not. Rarely is it necessary to use an armholding or suspension device; instead, have the assistant surgeon position the extremity. The distention is extremely important.

Enter the joint laterally with a 21-gauge needle. Palpate the radial capitular joint and identify it with pronation and supination. Inject saline into the joint at a point just anterior to the lateral epicondyle and just superior to the radial head. Maximal distention is essential, especially for posterior inspection. A posterolateral portal is used to inspect the olecranon fossa (Fig. 5-1). When the joint is distended maximally, note the bulge between the humerus and ulna. Make a stab wound over the bulge. Triangulation is possible from a posteromedial portal, but take care to avoid the ulnar nerve.

The anterior compartment can be approached either from a lateral or a medial aspect. The lateral approach is more frequently used. With adequate distention, palpate the radial capitular joint. Insert the scope just above the radial head and just anterior to the lateral epicondyle where saline was injected (Fig. 5-2). In this way, the anterior compartment can be inspected (Fig. 5-3). The medial approach for the arthroscope is just anterior and superior to the medial epicondyle.

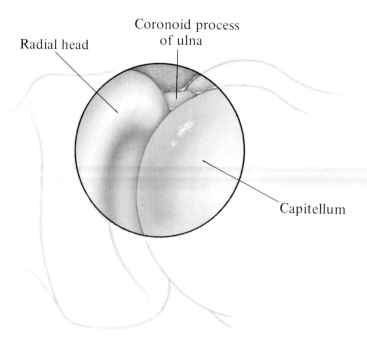

FIGURE 5-3. Lateral portal view.

References

1. Johnson, LL: *Diagnostic and Surgical Arthroscopy. The Knee and Other Joints.* St. Louis, Mosby, 1981, pp. 390–399.
2. Mital MA, Karlin LI: Diagnostic arthroscopy in sports injuries. *Orthop Clin North Am* 1980;11:771–785.
3. Andrews JR, Carson WG: Arthroscopy of the elbow. *Arthroscopy* 1985;1:97–107.

Additional Reading

Eriksson E, Sebik A. Arthroscopy and arthroscopic surgery in a gas versus fluid medium. *Orthop Clin North Am* 1982;13:293–298.

McGinty JB: Arthroscopic removal of loose bodies. *Orthop Clin North Am* 1982;13:313–328.

Renstrom P: Swedish research in sports traumatology. *Clin Orthop* 1984;191:144–158.

Lateral Epicondyle Release

6

H. Royer Collins

General Considerations

In most instances, lateral epicondylitis is treated successfully by conservative measures. However, surgical intervention is sometimes indicated in unrelenting cases. Many procedures have been advocated for relief of this symptom complex.[1,2] We prefer a relatively simple approach to this problem: lateral epicondylar release under local anesthesia.[3]

Surgical Procedure and Techniques

Prep the patient's arm and drape it in the usual fashion; apply a tourniquet to the upper extremity. Next, infiltrate local anesthetic into the skin after the exact point of tenderness has been determined by palpation. All that is necessary to give the desired exposure for this procedure is usually a small incision (2.5 cm–3 cm). Center this incision over the lateral epicondyle and the point of maximum tenderness (Fig. 6-1). Carry the dissection down to the lateral epicondyle and to the fascia overlying it and insert Senn retractors. At this time, carry out further palpation of the structures exposed. It is possible to determine the exact point of tenderness. Next, after further injection of local anesthetic, make a longitudinal incision directly over the point of maximum tenderness (Fig. 6-2). Usually, we are able to find an area of grayish granulation tissue deep to the extensor tendon, which is generally in the area

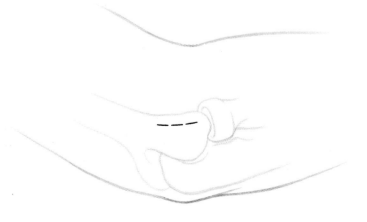

FIGURE 6-1

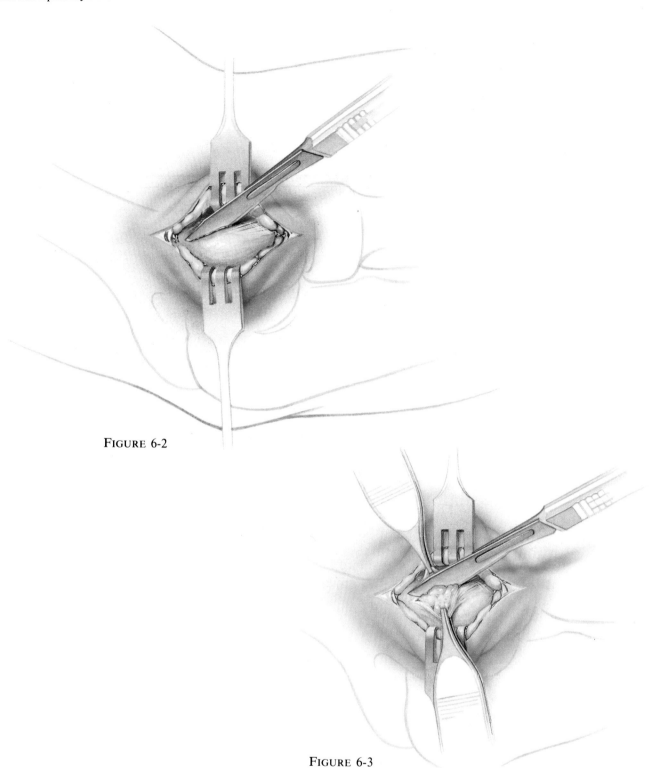

FIGURE 6-2

FIGURE 6-3

of the extensor carpi radialis brevis muscle. This incision is usually no longer than 1 cm in length from the lateral epicondyle.

Excise the area of degeneration (Fig. 6-3). Release the extensor carpi radialis brevis from its lateral epicondylar origin; after this is accomplished, a 5-mm gap is usually appreciated. Finally, roughen the lateral epicondyle using a sharp curette so that adequate new bleeding can be achieved (Fig. 6-4).

Close the fascia with Dexon suture and close the subcutaneous tissue with Dexon and the skin with a 4–0 clear nylon subcuticular stitch. Apply Steri-strips and a compression-type dressing before releasing the tourniquet.

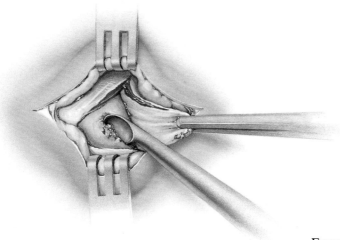

FIGURE 6-4

Postoperative Care and Rehabilitation

Postoperatively, allow the patient activity as his symptoms permit. Advise him against heavy weightlifting, but permit normal use of the hand as soon as pain subsides. By 3 weeks after surgery, it is usually time to institute a rehabilitation program of weightlifting (see Chap. 11). As soon as an adequate strength is achieved, the patient can return to athletic activity.

References

1. Boyd HB, McCleod AC: Tennis elbow. *J Bone Jt Surg* 1973;55A:1183–1187.
2. Posch JN, Goldberg VM, et al: Extensor fasciotomy for tennis elbow. *Clin Orthop* 1978;135:179–182.
3. Baumgard SH, Schwartz OR: Percutaneous release of the epicondylar muscles for humeral epicondylitis. *Am J Sports Med* 1982;10:233–236.

Additional Reading

Heyes-Moore GH: Resistant tennis elbow. *J Hand Surg* 1984;9:64–66.
Priest JD, Jones HH, Tichenor CJ, Nagael DA: Arm and elbow changes in expert tennis players. *Minn Med* 1977;60(5):399–404.
Rosen JM, Duffy FP, Miller EH, Kremchek EJ: Tennis elbow syndrome: Results of the "lateral release" procedure. *Ohio State Med J.* 1980;76(2):103–109.

7

Debridement

James E. Tibone and H. Royer Collins

General Considerations

Loose bodies form in the elbow as a result of osteochondritis dissecans or as a result of repetitive trauma caused by the radial head compressing against the capitellum and the olecranon impinging into the olecranon fossa. This repetitive trauma, with hypertrophy of the distal end of the humerus and of the tip of the olecranon, leads to a poor fit in the olecranon fossa and predisposes to articular cartilage damage.[1-3]

Surgery to remove the loose bodies in the elbow should be done through an incision that will allow as normal a recovery of function as possible. The fullness of recovery depends on three factors: dissecting between planes of muscles so that early return of motion can be accomplished; removing the loose bodies; and correcting the incongruity of the olecranon in the olecranon fossa.

Surgical Procedure and Techniques

Surgery is accomplished with a tourniquet applied to the upper extremity while the patient is in a supine position and the arm is draped free. Start the incision approximately 3 cm proximal to the lateral epicondyle in line with the lateral border of the humerus and the triceps. Extend it distally over the lateral epicondyle while curving it between the radial head and the ulna (Fig. 7-1).

Develop the interval between the anconeus muscle and the extensor carpi ulnaris muscle and expose the underlying elbow capsule. Then, open the capsule of the radioulnar joint with a longitudinal incision and inspect the joint (Fig. 7-2).

Loose bodies can usually be removed through the small incision, but it may be necessary, at times, to "T" the capsule anteriorly to give wider exposure. In this case, carry the incision up proximally along the epicondylar ridge until the triceps is identified. Then, with sharp dissection, displace the triceps posteriorly to expose the tip of the olecranon and the olecranon fossa. This maneuver will allow loose bodies to be removed from this area.

Once this is accomplished, remove the tip of the olecranon with a ¼-inch osteotome (Fig. 7-3). This osteotomy should be carried out just proximal to the insertion of the triceps tendon. Then, smooth the tip of the olecranon

FIGURE 7-1

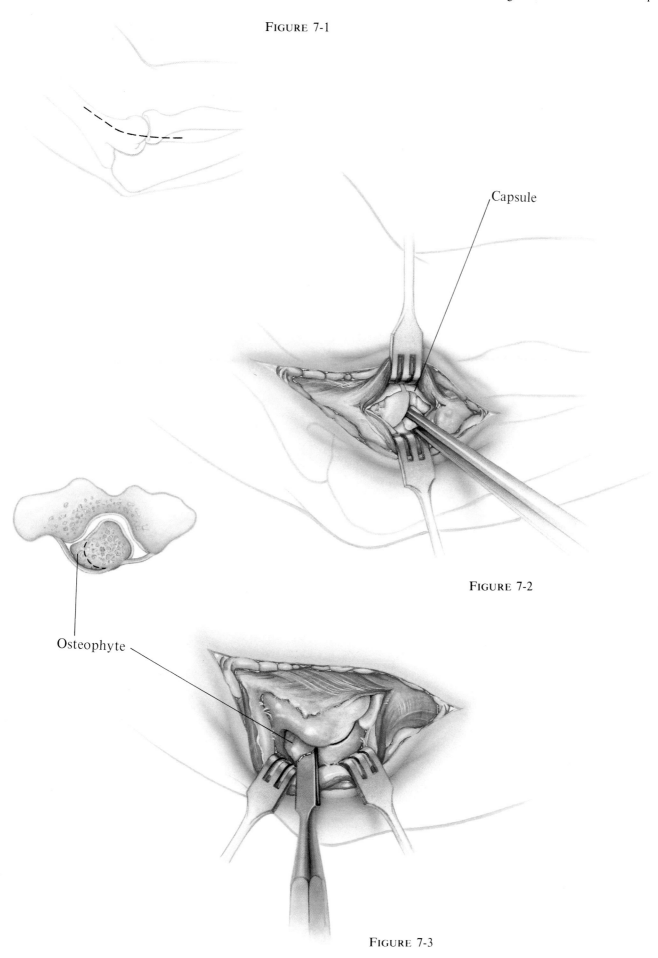

Capsule

FIGURE 7-2

Osteophyte

FIGURE 7-3

with a rongeur. When using the rongeur and osteotome, avoid going too far medially and thus damaging the ulnar nerve. Wider exposure can be obtained through this incision by placing a varus stress on the elbow joint.

After thorough irrigation, close the capsule with a #2–0 Dexon suture; close the interval between the epicondylar ridge and the triceps by using this same suture. Next, close the anconeus and the extensor carpi ulnaris fascia, again by using #2–0 Dexon suture. Finally, close the subcutaneous tissue with #3–0 Dexon suture, followed by subcuticular clear #4–0 nylon to close the skin. Steri-strips and a compression-type dressing are next applied with the arm immobilized in approximately 90 degrees of flexion with a posterior molded plaster splint.

Postoperative Care and Rehabilitation

At the end of the first postoperative week, remove the splint and start an early range of motion exercises. At 3 weeks, start a strengthening program and begin rehabilitation for full return to athletic activities as outlined in Chapter 11. At 3 months postoperatively, the athlete can usually return to his sport.

References

1. Wilson FD, Andrews JR, Blackburn TA, McCluskey G: Valgus extension overload in the pitching elbow. *Am J Sports Med* 1983;11:83–88.
2. Woodward AH, Bianco AJ: Osteochondritis dissecans of the elbow. *Clin Orthop* 1975;110:35–41.
3. Brown R, Blazina ME, et al: Osteochondritis of the capitellum. *J Sports Med* 1974;2:27–46.

Additional Reading

McManama GB Jr, Micheli LJ, Berry MV, Sohn RS: The surgical treatment of osteochondritis of the capitellum. *Am J Sports Med* 1985;13:11–21.

Pappas AM: Osteochondritis dissecans. *Clin Orthop* 1981;158:59–69.

Priest JD, Weise DJ: Elbow injury in women's gymnastics. *Am J Sports Med* 1981;9:288–295.

Tivnon MC, Anzel SH, Waugh TR: Surgical management of osteochondritis dissecans of the capitellum. *Am J Sports Med* 1976;4:121–128.

Medial Collateral Ligament Reconstruction

8

H. Royer Collins and Clarence L. Shields, Jr.

General Considerations

Occasionally, in the act of throwing or in other sports requiring forceful valgus stress at the elbow, rupture of the medial or ulnar collateral ligament of the elbow may occur.[1,2] The athlete is usually aware of a sudden sharp pain in the medial side of the elbow and frequently feels a tearing or hears a pop similar to the symptoms associated with tear of the medial collateral ligament of the knee joint. There is usually immediate disability. Upon examination, the patient presents with no stability in the medial side of the joint. Under valgus stress, there is an opening of the joint on the medial side.[3] Also, there is usually tenderness at the site of the injury. This injury may be associated with ulnar nerve symptoms as a result of the trauma that has occurred. In chronic cases, gravity stress films are positive and the reconstruction of the medial collateral ligament is necessary.

Surgical Procedure and Techniques

The repair is carried out with the same approach that is used for transfer of the ulnar nerve (Fig. 8-1). Incise the flexor muscle mass at its origin at the epicondyle and retract it distally (Fig. 8-2). Retract the ulnar nerve out of harms way to expose the medial collateral ligament, medial epicondyle, and the medial surface of the olecranon, including the tubercle on the coracoid process. Cut a notch in the intermuscular spetum for the ulnar nerve transfer. Place two drill holes approximately 1.0 cm apart through the medial epicondyle

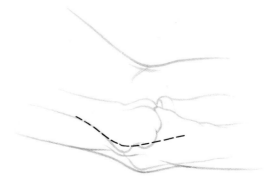

FIGURE 8-1

49

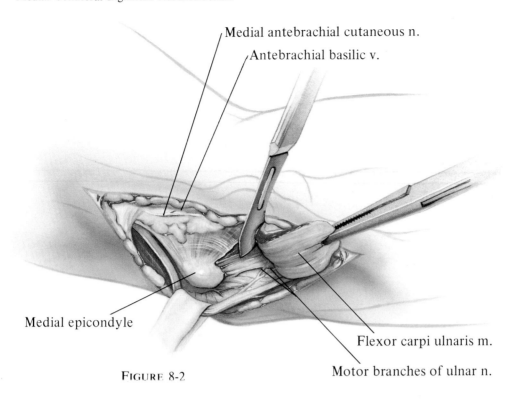

Medial antebrachial cutaneous n.

Antebrachial basilic v.

Medial epicondyle

Flexor carpi ulnaris m.

Motor branches of ulnar n.

FIGURE 8-2

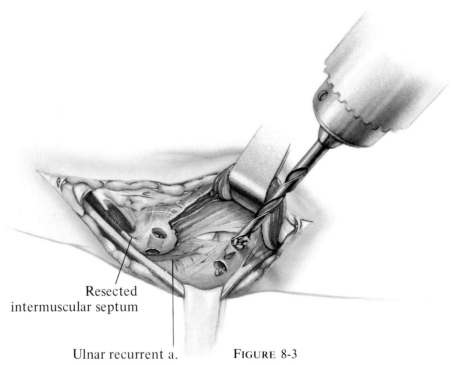

Resected
intermuscular septum

Ulnar recurrent a.

FIGURE 8-3

to form a bone tunnel. Next, place two similar drill holes in the olecranon at its usual insertion of the medial collateral ligament (Fig. 8-3).

Now, turn attention to the opposite forearm; and drape it so that the palmaris longus muscle can be removed from this forearm. It is preferable to take the palmaris longus from the nondominant arm in the throwing athlete so that the weakness is less likely to occur in active throwing.

It is obviously essential to be certain that the patient does have a palmaris longus muscle present in this arm since it may be absent in a significant percentage of patients. Make 2 cm incision in the flexor crease at the wrist

50

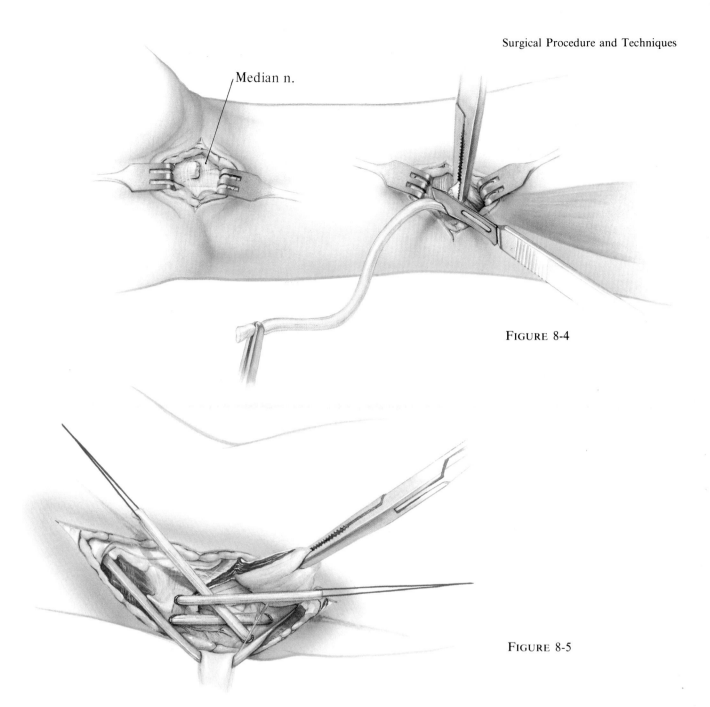

Median n.

FIGURE 8-4

FIGURE 8-5

to expose the palmar fascia and the palmaris longus muscle as it inserts into this palmar fascia. Take care not to go too deep since the median nerve generally lies just deep to this. Sometimes, however, it is off to either side and can be easily injured in the act of harvesting the palmaris longus tendon.

Grasp the tendon and make a second incision parallel to this incision approximately 7.5 cm proximal to the first incision (Fig. 8-4). The palmaris longus tendon is exposed at this level. Next, transect it at its distal level with a sharp #10 blade and pull it proximally to exit from the proximal wound. Then transect the tendon near its insertion after giving it as much length as can be achieved. Close these incisions and use the harvested palmaris longus tendon as a substitute for the medial collateral ligament.

Place a Bunnell type suture of #1 Ethibond in one end of the tendon to facilitate its passage through the bone tunnels. Now, bring the palmaris longus tendon first through the anterior drill hole at the medial epicondyle, next distally through the posterior drill hole in the epicondyle, and then distally through the anterior hole in the olecranon (Fig. 8-5). A figure-8 pattern will

51

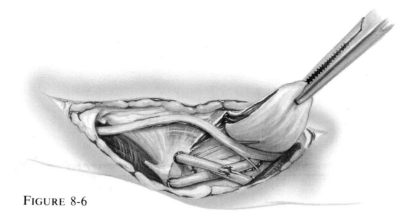

FIGURE 8-6

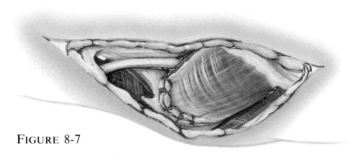

FIGURE 8-7

be produced. Suture the two ends of the tendon together with #1 Ethibond in an overlapping fashion under good tension to recreate a medial collateral ligament (Fig. 8-6). Finally, transfer the ulnar nerve deep to the flexor muscle mass. Always resect a small portion of the intermuscular septum prior to reattaching the flexor tendon to its origin in the medial epicondyle (Fig. 8-7). Close the incision with #0 Vicryl; as in the surgery for the ulnar nerve transfer, apply a posterior plaster splint.

Postoperative Care and Rehabilitation

It is necessary to protect the elbow for approximately a 6-week period of time until there is good union of the ligament, although controlled early motion is advisable to prevent limitation of motion (Chap. 11).

References

1. Norwood LA, Shook JA, et al: Acute elbow ruptures *Am J Sports Med* 1981;9:16–19.
2. Indelicato PA, Jobe FW, et al: Correctable elbow lesions in professional baseball players: A review of 25 cases. *Am J Sports Med* 1979;7:72–75.
3. Schwab GH, Bennett JB, Woods GW: Biomechanics of elbow instability: The role of the medial collateral ligament. *Clin Orthop* 1980;146:42–52.

Additional Reading

Dehaven KE, Evarts CM: Throwing injuries of the elbow in athletes. *Ortho Clin North Am* 1973;4:801–808.

Ulnar Nerve Transfer

9

H. Royer Collins

General Considerations

Irritation of the ulnar nerve frequently occurs in the athlete who throws. This irritation manifests itself in tenderness at the elbow and occasionally causes a radiation of symptoms into the fourth and fifth fingers.[2] With activity, the nerve may also sublux in the groove and produce tenderness there. Often there is a positive Tinel's sign.

If symptoms do not respond to the usual conservative management, surgery may be indicated. In our experience, subcutaneous transfer of the ulnar nerve is not adequate, and it has been necessary to transfer the ulnar nerve deep to the flexor muscle mass.[1,3]

Surgical Procedure and Techniques

Place the patient either under general anesthesia or brachial block anesthesia and apply a tourniquet to the upper arm. Throughout the procedure, the patient is supine with the arm on an armboard. Center the incision over the medial epicondyle, extending it approximately 5 cm proximal to the medial epicondyle, in line with the ulnar nerve. Then, course the incision distal from the medial epicondyle for a distance of 5 cm toward the ulnar crest (Fig. 9-1). Carry the dissection down through the fascia while taking care to avoid injury to the ulnar nerve. This dissection is posterior to the intermuscular septum between the brachialis and the triceps muscles. Be sure to carry the dissection far enough into this groove so that there is absolutely no evidence of impingement of the ulnar nerve. Then, follow the nerve in its groove, posterior to the medial condyle. Because the ulnar nerve in the groove is

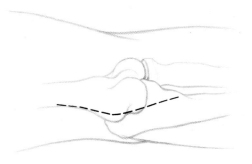

FIGURE 9-1

53

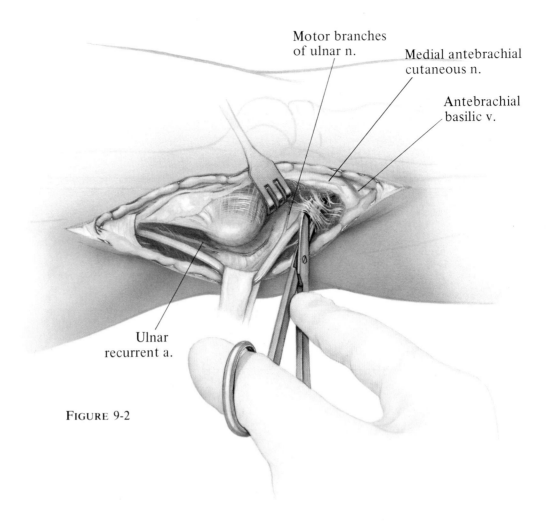

Motor branches
of ulnar n.

Medial antebrachial
cutaneous n.

Antebrachial
basilic v.

Ulnar
recurrent a.

FIGURE 9-2

accompanied by branches of the brachial artery, take great care to avoid
any injury to them. During this dissection, protect the ulnar nerve by using
either an umbilical tape or a PenRose drain. In most instances, there are
no branches of the ulnar nerve above the medial epicondyle, but because
occasionally there are, proceed with due caution.

Just distal to the medial epicondyle, the ulnar nerve begins to branch into
the flexor forearm musculature. Exercise care in dissecting these branches
free in order to have the nerve completely free to be transferred (Fig. 9-2).
Generally, dissection can be carried between the two heads of the flexor carpi
ulnaris. Because the recurrent ulnar artery follows the ulnar nerve in the
groove, take special care so that it is not damaged. If necessary, however,
in order to be able to mobilize the nerve well, this artery may have to be
ligated. Now release the origin of the flexor carpi ulnaris from the medial
epicondyle with sharp dissection. Leave the pronator teres untouched if possible so that no attention need be given to the median nerve that lies lateral
to it. Retract the flexor distally for a distance of approximately 2.5 cm (Fig.
9-3). This will allow enough room to transfer the ulnar nerve and to lay it
in a bed without too much kinking. Prior to transferring the ulnar nerve,
we generally resect a small portion of the intermusclar septum so that no
tight band will impinge against the ulnar nerve. This section of the intermuscular septum extends approximately 2.5 cm proximal to the medial epicondyle.
Now, bring the ulnar nerve out of its groove and place it just deep to the
flexor muscle mass. Next, bring the flexor muscle over the ulnar nerve and
reattach it to its origin with #0 Dexon sutures (Fig. 9-4).

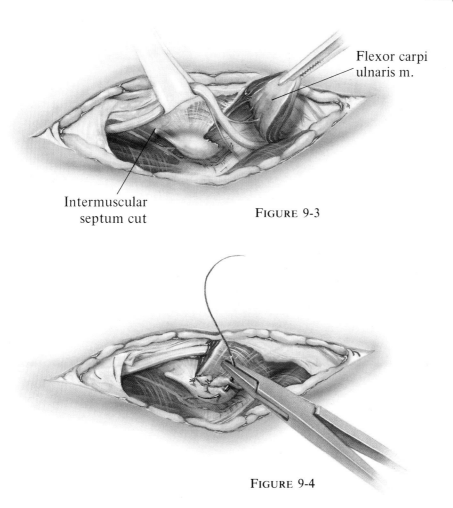

Flexor carpi
ulnaris m.

Intermuscular
septum cut

FIGURE 9-3

FIGURE 9-4

It may be necessary to make small drill holes into the epicondyle for acceptance of the sutures, but this is not always necessary. As we indicated above,
it is extremely important that there be no kinks in the ulnar nerve as it
passes through this submuscle tunnel.

Finally, close the fascial layer with interrupted Dexon sutures, close the
subcutaneous with interrupted Dexon sutures, and close the subcuticular layer
with nylon sutures. Place Steri-strips over the skin. With the elbow at 90
degrees and wrapped in a compression-type dressing, place the patient's arm
in a posterior plaster splint.

Postoperative Care and Rehabilitation

After keeping the patient in a posterior splint for 1 week, encourage a range
of active motion exercise. Do not permit excessive hand gripping, however,
until approximately 3 weeks after the surgery, when good fixation of the
flexor forearm musculature is usually achieved. When this point is reached,
have the patient carry out gradual rehabilitation of the forearm musculature
and, as symptoms allow, return to throwing activities (Chap. 11).

References

1. Del Pizzo W, Jobe FW, Norwood L: Ulnar entrapment syndrome in baseball
   players. *Am J Sports Med* 1977;5:182–185.
2. Indelicato PA, Jobe FW, et al: Correctable elbow lesions in professional baseball
   players: A review of 25 cases. *Am J Sports Med* 1979;7:72–75.

3. Posner MA: Submuscular transposition for the ulnar nerve at the elbow. *Bull Hosp Jt Dis Orthop Inst* 1984;44(2):406–423.

Additional Reading

Chan RC, Paine KW, Varughese G: Ulnar neuropathy at the elbow: Comparison of simple decompression and anterior transposition. *Neurosurgery* 1980;7:545–550.

Eaton RG, Crowe JF, Parkes JC: Anterior transposition of the ulnar nerve using a non-compressing fasciodermal sling. *J Bone Jt Surg* 1980;62A:820–825.

Foster RJ, Edshage S: Factors related to the outcome of surgically managed compressive ulnar neuropathy at the elbow level. *J Hand Surg* 1981;6:181–192.

Richmond JC, Southmayd WW: Superficial anterior transposition of the ulnar nerve at the elbow for ulnar neuritis. *Clin Orthop* 1982;164:42–44.

Repair of Distal Biceps Tendon Rupture

10

James E. Tibone

General Considerations

Ruptures of the biceps tendon from the radial tuberosity are uncommon, not rare. Such a rupture usually occurs in weightlifters or bodybuilders. It may also occur in the elderly population, but these patients need no treatment.[1] Surgical repair of the biceps tendon is essential in the weightlifter or bodybuilder to restore the full strength of elbow flexion and forearm supination.[2,4]

In addition, the cosmetic deformity that results from the proximal retraction of the biceps muscle is not acceptable to the bodybuilder. The results of surgery usually provide return of full function to the upper extremity.

Surgical Procedure and Techniques

Place the patient supine on the operating table with the arm on a conventional handboard. Use a modification of the two-incision technique as described by Boyd and Anderson.[3] The incidence of radial nerve palsy is high when a one-incision approach is used.

Make an oblique incision approximately 1 to 2 cm above the elbow crease just medial to the biceps tendon (Fig. 10-1). Curve the incision across the elbow crease approximately 1 to 2 cm distal to the elbow joint. This maneuver gives a more cosmetic scar than the conventional S-incision as described by Boyd and Anderson.[3] The cutaneous terminal branch of the musculocutaneous

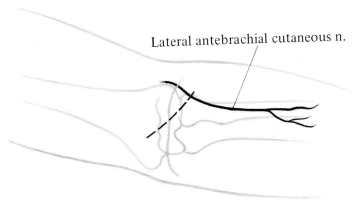

Lateral antebrachial cutaneous n.

FIGURE 10-1

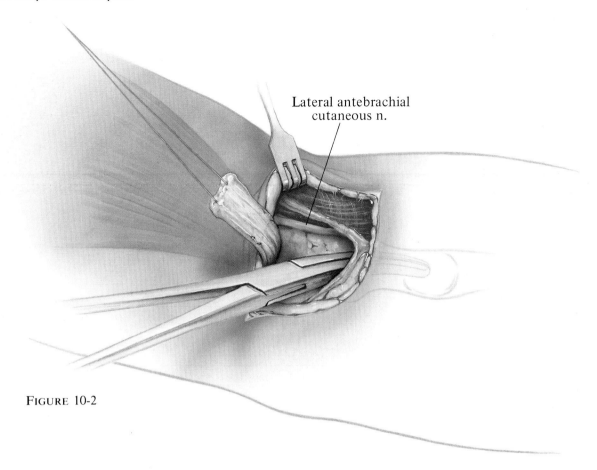

Lateral antebrachial
cutaneous n.

FIGURE 10-2

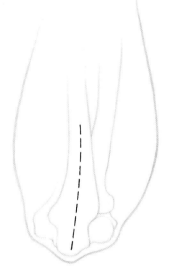

FIGURE 10-3. Posterior incision is made while forearm is supinated.

nerve lies just lateral to the biceps tendon and must be protected. To avoid the nerve, carry out the dissection either anterior or just medial to the biceps muscle. Divide the fascia overlying the anterior aspect of the arm to expose the ruptured tendon, which is usually retracted approximately 3 to 5 cm above the elbow joint. Freshen the end of the tendon and weave a Bunnell-type suture through the end of the tendon with a #1 Ethibond suture. With a curved clamp, locate the tunnel between the radius and ulna by blunt dissection (Fig. 10-2). It is not necessary to dissect the anterior aspect of the elbow.

Now, flex the elbow and turn your attention to the posterior aspect of the extremity. Make an incision that is 8 to 12 cm along the subcutaneous border of the ulna and that extends from the tip of the olecranon distally (Fig. 10-3). Elevate the muscles along the lateral aspect of the proximal ulna and retract them laterally. This includes the supinator muscle, which is lying deep, and overlying the radial head and neck. (The radial nerve is still anterior to the elbow and is protected by the spinator muscle and is not in danger of injury.)

Now, pronate the forearm, allowing the radial tuberosity to be palpated and cleared of soft tissue. Next, drill a hole through the outer cortex of the bicipital tuberosity (Fig. 10-4). Do this with an ⅛-inch and then a ¼-inch drill bit and enlarge the holes with rongeurs and curettes to make a tunnel for the tendon. On the opposite side of the tuberosity, drill two small holes with a 5/64-inch drill bit. Pass the tendon from the anterior incision through the tunnel between the radius and ulna into the posterior incision.

At this point, it is important to close the anterior incision since this becomes difficult once the elbow is flexed after the tendon becomes fixed to the radial tuberosity. After the subcutaneous tissue and skin are closed on the anterior

58

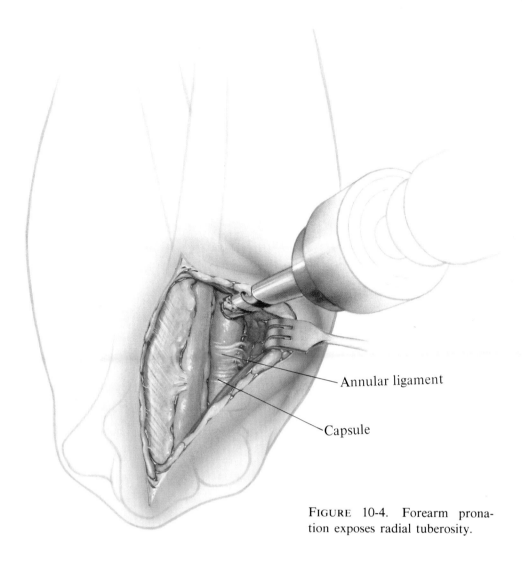

Annular ligament

Capsule

FIGURE 10-4. Forearm pronation exposes radial tuberosity.

incision, pass the sutures into the tunnel and out the small drill holes. This
is the most difficult aspect of the operation.

The easiest method of suturing is to pass a loop of 24-gauge wire through
the small drill hole into the tunnel and to pull the Ethibond suture back
with the wire (Fig. 10-5). When both sutures have been passed and the tendon
is in the tunnel, tie the suture after flexing the elbow 90 degrees and placing
the forearm in supination (Fig. 10-6). If the tendon is seated in the bone, it
is usually not necessary to place any reinforcing sutures.

Reattach the muscles that have been elevated to the proximal ulna and
close the subcutaneous tissue and skin in a routine fashion. Finally, immobilize
the patient in mediolateral and posterior splints with the elbow flexed 90
degrees and the forearm in supination. When the swelling subsides, immobilize
the patient's extremity in a long arm cast for a total of 6 weeks.

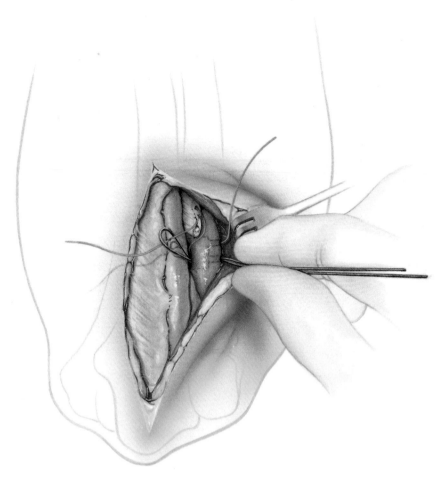

FIGURE 10-5. Forearm is supinated for suture retrieval.

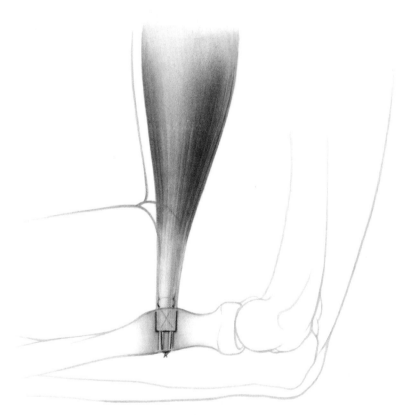

FIGURE 10-6. Forearm supinated.

Postoperative Care and Rehabilitation

Following removal of the cast at the end of 6 weeks of postoperative recovery, start the patient on a gentle active range of motion. Avoid all passive exercises and permit no weights for the first 6 weeks out of the cast. By this time, the patient has usually recovered most of his motion, although the last few degrees of extension may be lacking. At 12 weeks postoperatively, start the patient on a gentle weight program with isometric and isotonic exercises, but do not permit any heavy weights for another 12 weeks. At 6 months postoperatively, the athlete can usually begin his training for weightlifting or bodybuilding competition, although it may take an additional 3 to 6 months for him to reach a competitive level.

References

1. Baker BE: Operative vs. non-operative treatments of disruption of the distal tendon of biceps. *Orthop Rev* 1982;11(10):71.
2. Baker BE, Bierwagen D: Rupture of the distal tendon of the biceps brachii: Operative versus non-operative treatment. *J Bone Jt Surg* 1985;67A:414–417.
3. Boyd HB, Anderson LD: A method for reinsertion of the distal biceps brachii tendon. *J Bone Jt Surg* 1961;43A:1041–1043.
4. Hovelius L, Josefsson G: Rupture of the distal biceps tendon. Report of five cases. *Acta Orthop Scand* 1977;48(3):280–282.

Additional Reading

Del Pizzo W, Norwood LA, et al: Rupture of the biceps tendon in gymnastics; a case report. *Am J Sports Med* 1978;6:283–286.

Morrey BF, Askey LJ, et al: Rupture of the distal tendon of the biceps brachii; a biomechanical study. *J Bone Jt Surg* 1985;67:418–421.

Norman WH: Repair of avulsion of insertion of biceps brachii tendon. *Clin Orthop* 1985;193:189–194.

Postacchini F, Puddu G: Subcutaneous rupture of the distal biceps brachii tendon: A report of seven cases. J Sports Med 1975;15:81–90.

Vastamaeki M, Brummer H, Soloner KA: Avulsion of the distal biceps brachii tendon. *Acta Orthop Scan* 1981;52(1):45–58.

11 Rehabilitation of the Upper Extremity

Clive E. Brewster, Clarence L. Shields, Jr.,
Judy L. Seto, and Matthew C. Morrissey

Determining Rehabilitative Goals

In throwing and racquet sports, the dominant shoulder is usually the stronger and more flexible shoulder. An important factor in determinig the treatment goals is the level of competition the patient aspires to. An equally important factor, especially in team sports, is the specific playing position that the athlete holds since the type and amount of shoulder movement required will differ depending on that position. For example, in football the type and amount needed by a quarterback is quite different from that needed by an offensive lineman.

Before attempting to work out a rehabilitative program, obtain the details of the surgical procedure and any precautions noted by the surgeon. Within this context, first test the active range of motion by assessing several variables: the patient's willingness to move, the quality of motion displayed, the scapulo-humeral rhythm, and the presence of any painful arcs through the range of movement. Record the active range of motion for both shoulders. Flexion, extension, abduction, internal and external rotation, and horizontal abduction and adduction are measured with a goniometer placed at the glenohumeral joint's axis of rotation. It is important to observe the scapulohumeral rhythm posteriorly to determine any abnormalities during flexion and abduction.

The range of tests for active motion assess the contractile structures (e.g., muscles); the range of tests for passive motion gauge the influence of both contractile and noncontractile tissues on the extremity's motion (e.g., the joint capsule and ligaments and the articular cartilage surfaces). By testing the ranges of active and passive motion, one can demonstrate the degree of joint hypomobility or of hypermobility.

Basic Rehabilitation Protocol: The Shoulder

The Starting Phase

Warmup

In general, the early stages of rehabilitation consist of therapy to relieve pain and stiffness while restoring motion. Pain, which usually presents as a general aching complaint, can be reduced by applying 10 to 15 minutes of heat (e.g.,

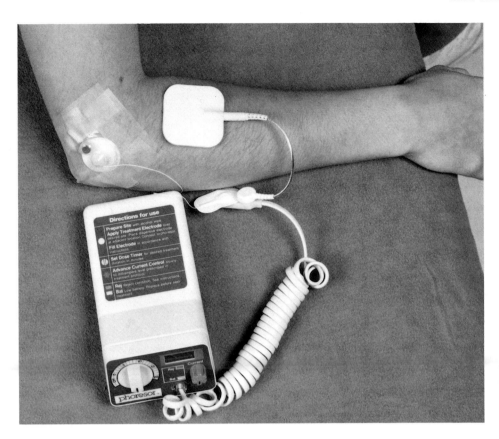

FIGURE 11-1. Iontophoresis: Elbow. (Phoresor model PM 600; Motion Control, Inc., Salt Lake City, UT 84101).

moist hotpacks) and then 10 to 15 minutes of cold (e.g., icepacks) after the heat treatment. The use of the heat-and-cold contrast acts as a physiological pump to decrease inflammation and to stimulate circulation in the shoulder.[2,4]

For the treatment of pain, transcutaneous electrical stimulation can also be used to provide an afferent nerve block. Two other modalities that may be used to decrease both pain and inflammation are iontophoresis and phonophoresis. Iontophoresis is the introduction of ions of medication into the tissue by means of direct current. When using the phoresor, the placement of the electrode is extremely important. Although a number of medications can be used, we prefer to use 1 cc Hexadrol and 2 cc of 4 percent viscous Xylocaine mixed into a gel. This works well when the area treated is superficial approximately 1 to 2 inches deep (Fig. 11-1). Phonophoresis is the introduction of medication into the tissue by means of ultrasound. We use 1 cc of Hexadrol and 1 cc of 4 percent Xylocaine mixed in with a small amount of ultrasound gel. Depending on the intensity of the ultrasound, this modality penetrates deeper into the tissue than does iontophoresis (Fig. 11-2).

Stretches

Because of the immobilization that is mandatory after surgery, most surgical patients present with diffuse shoulder hypomobility. Based on the findings of the active and passive motion components of the initial evaluation, treatment will include physiological stretching. Each stretch produces gentle movement of the humeral head against the glenoid. Have the patient hold the position for 10 to 20 seconds and follow it by a 10-second relaxation period. For each stretch, the patient should perform two sets of 10 repetitions.

Shoulder Internal and External Rotation Stretches. Place the patient in a standing position and have her hold the arm in the anatomical position (Fig.

63

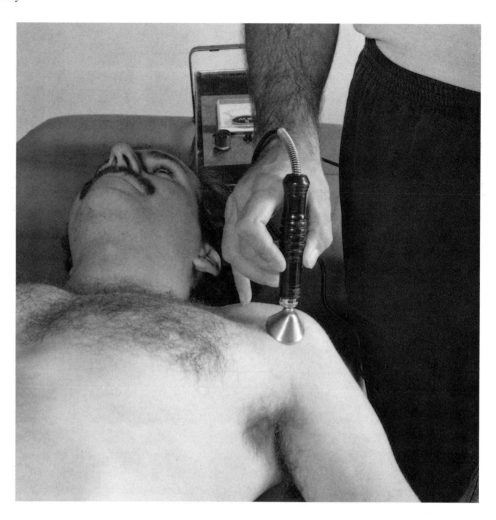

FIGURE 11-2. Phonophoresis: Shoulder.

11-3A). Then have her smoothly rotate the arm into external rotation in order to stretch the anterior capsule. This movement will also gently elongate posterior shoulder structures by the internal humeral rotation (Fig. 11-3B).

Saw Exercises.   Have the patient stand or sit with the shoulder in an anatomical position and the elbow flexed to 90 degrees (Fig. 11-4). Then have her move the shoulder back and forth from extension to flexion. This movement will flex the elbow in shoulder extension and extend it in shoulder flexion. The movements of shoulder extension and flexion help to reeducate the patient in shoulder movement.

Cross-Body Saw Exercises.   The patient positions the elbow in 90 degrees of flexion and internally rotates the arm (Fig. 11-5A). The arm is adducted and abducted as the arm is brought across the front of the body (Fig. 11-5B). These exercises are utilized to gain shoulder abduction and adduction motion.

Pendulum Exercises.   This exercise is most easily performed while standing with feet approximately shoulder width apart and hips flexed to 90 degress. The knees are slightly bent allowing the involved arm to hang loosely in a relaxed position. The unaffected arm may hold onto a stable object (e.g., table or chair) for support. From this position the trunk moves in a slow rhythmical fashion causing the arm to swing freely like a pendulum. Have the patient hold a 2-pound weight for additional traction (Fig. 11-6). To get

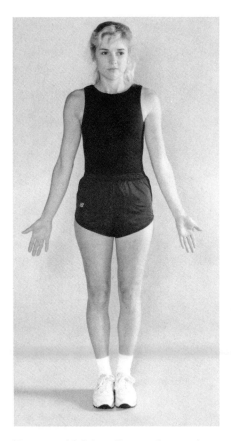

FIGURE 11-3A. External rotation stretch: Shoulder.

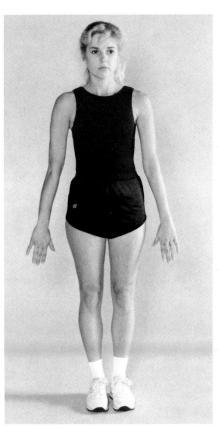

FIGURE 11-3B. Internal rotation stretch: Shoulder.

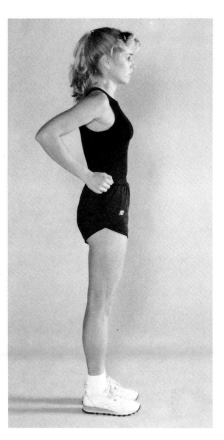

FIGURE 11-4. Saw exercise: Shoulder.

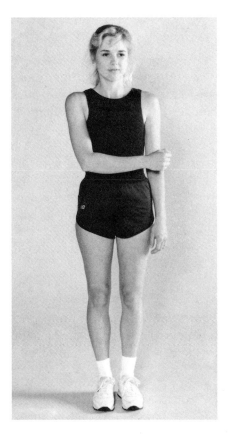

FIGURE 11-5A. Cross-body saw exercise: Shoulder

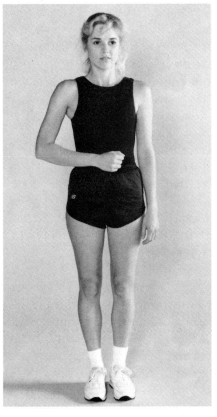

FIGURE 11-5B. Cross-body saw exercise: Shoulder

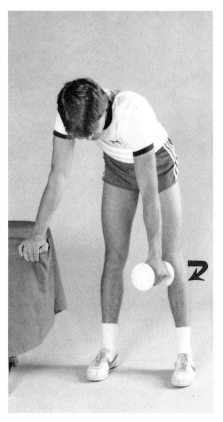

FIGURE 11-6. Pendulum exercise: Shoulder

65

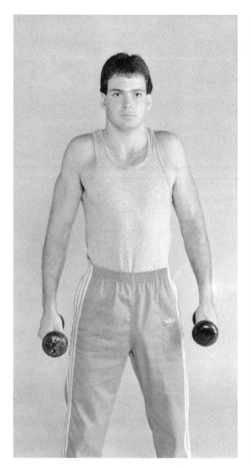 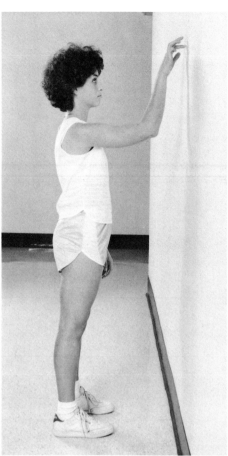

FIGURE 11-7. Shrug exercise: Shoulder.

FIGURE 11-8. Wall-slide flexion exercise: Shoulder.

FIGURE 11-7   FIGURE 11-8

full value from this exercise, have the patient start with small circles in a clockwise direction and gradually increase the diameter of the circle. Have the patient perform two sets of 10 repetitions and then switch to counterclockwise rotation for the same number of exercises. This set of exercises provides a gentle traction force that helps relax the shoulder joint muscles. In addition, this exercise distracts the humeral head from the glenoid fossa.

Shoulder Shrug Exercises. Shoulder shrugs are initially performed with the patient standing, arms extended, and holding the wand in front of the body. To have the patient progress in these exercises, have him hold a 2-pound weight in each hand (Fig. 11-7). Next, have him elevate the shoulders and lower them in a circular fashion. This motion incoporates shoulder protraction/retraction to maintain mobility in the scapulothoracic, sternoclavicular, and acromioclavicular joints.

Wall Slide Exercises. The patient executes wall slides while standing and facing the wall for flexion. By using a wall to support the hand in an upward movement of the shoulder into flexion, the patient places less stress on the injured shoulder. Have the patient "finger walk" the hand up the wall into flexion while slowly moving the rest of the body closer to the wall. When the end of range is reached, have the patient hold this stretch position for 5 seconds (Fig. 11-8) and then slowly "walk" the hand back down the wall while gradually moving the body away from it.

For an abduction stretch, have the patient stand with the injured shoulder closest to the wall and repeat the climbing in this new position (Fig. 11-9).

66

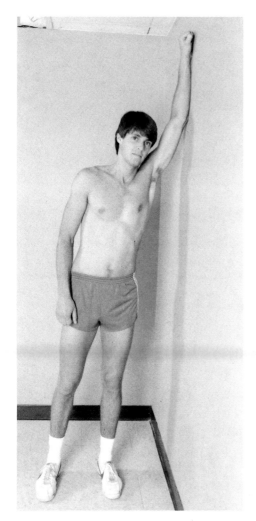

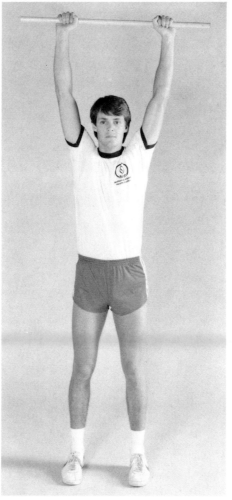

FIGURE 11-9. Abduction stretch: Shoulder.

FIGURE 11-10. Wand flexion exercise: Shoulder.

FIGURE 11-9   FIGURE 11-10

This exercise does two things: it offers stretching at the end of the range of motion; it allows the shoulder muscles—those that are responsible for shoulder flexion and abduction—to contract at ranges of motion that are unattainable without the assistance of a wall.

Wand Exercises.   Next, have the patient stand and perform wand exercises. These begin by having the patient grasp a wand with both hands. Although these exercises will eventually allow him to perform all the motions of the shoulder, he must approach this stage by easy steps. First, to accomplish flexion, have the patient grasp the stick with both hands and stretch both arms straight out in front of the abdomen. With the elbows extended, the patient then elevates the stick as high as possible (Fig. 11-10) and then slowly lowers it to the starting position. He performs two sets of 10 repetitions.

While in the supine position, the patient can perform mild adduction and abduction by moving the wand from side in front of the body. For more abduction, the patient can place the hand on the injured side at the end of the stick (Fig. 11-11). She controls the motion with the normal hand, which grasps the wand. Have her execute two sets of 10 repetitions.

To achieve internal and external rotation, have the patient hold the stick anterior to the abdomen and flex the elbows at 90 degrees while holding them in close contact with the rib cage. Then have the patient move the stick from left to right to provide shoulder rotation.

67

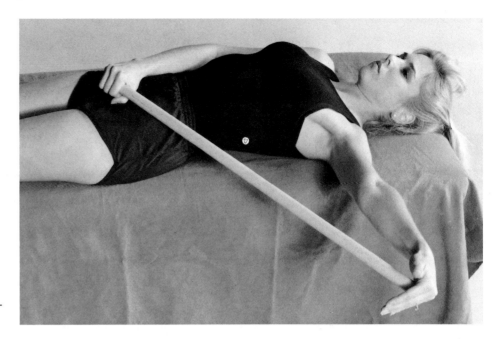

FIGURE 11-11. Wand abduction exercise: Shoulder.

Joint Mobilization

The focus of glenohumeral mobilization early in rehabilitation is conservative. The goals of returning joint motion and decreasing pain and soreness are foremost in this subacute stage. Four grades of movement are used to treat pain and stiffness and encompass the joint's available range of motion (Fig. 11-12). Grades I and II are used to decrease pain and are initiated at the beginning of the range of motion. Grade I is a small amplitude movement, while Grade II is a large amplitude oscillation within the range. Neither Grade I or II is to the end of the range. In treating stiffness or limited motion, Grades III and IV are used. The Grade III movement consists of large amplitude oscillations performed to the end of the range. Grade IV is a small amplitude movement at the end of the range. Long axis traction, lateral distraction, and caudal glides are commonly used mobilization techniques that offer a generalized stretch of the joint capsule and help relax the surrounding musculature.[14]

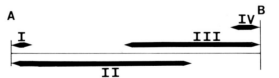

FIGURE 11-12. Joint mobilization stages.

Another motion that should be emphasized is caudal glides to decrease hypomobility. This motion is especially necessary after a period of shoulder immobility in the neutral position.

In addition to accessory mobilization, careful physiological mobilization into all the planes of motion may be started soon after surgery.[1] The usual emphasis is on external rotation, abduction, and flexion because they are the more functional motions of the glenohumeral joint and also because they are commonly affected by the period of surgery and immobility.

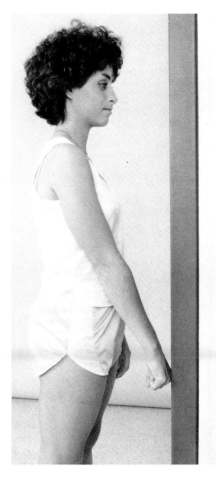 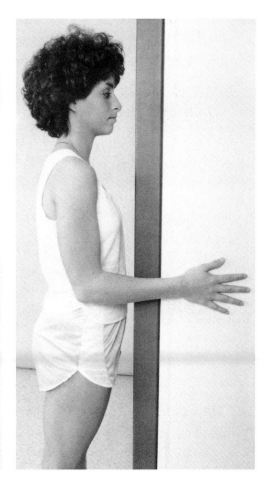

FIGURE 11-13. Isometric flex-ion exercise: Shoulder.

FIGURE 11-14. Isometric in-ternal rotation exercise: Shoul-der.

FIGURE 11-13   FIGURE 11-14

Isometric Exercises

Isometric exercises are performed to strengthen the muscles used in flexion, extension, abduction, and internal/external rotation. All the exercises begin with the shoulder in neutral position and the patient standing adjacent to a wall. For shoulder flexion, the patient faces the wall with the arms at her side and extends the elbow on the involved side. In this position, the dorsal surface of the hand is pushed forward against the wall with a maximal contraction (Fig. 11-13). The muscle is held taut for 10 seconds and then relaxed for 5 seconds. The athlete will do two sets of 10 repetitions with a 2-minute rest period between sets.

In isometric extension, she stands with her back against the wall. The arm is held in extension and the palm and arm are pushed against the wall.

To work the shoulder in abduction, she merely turns sideways to the wall and pushes the back of the hand and arm against the wall. Internal rotation is performed with the elbow flexed to 90 degrees and held close to the body. The patient stands in a doorway and attempts to rotate the forearm internally against the door jam (Fig. 11-14). For external rotation, she pushes the forearm outwardly against the opposite side of the entryway.

Home Program

The patient performs the same stretches at home as in therapy. He maintains the same number of sets and repetitions after being instructed how to use ice for 10 to 15 minutes after each workout period. Isometric exercises are performed with the shoulder in the neutral position.

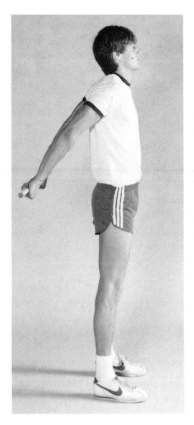

FIGURE 11-15. Extension stretch: Shoulder.

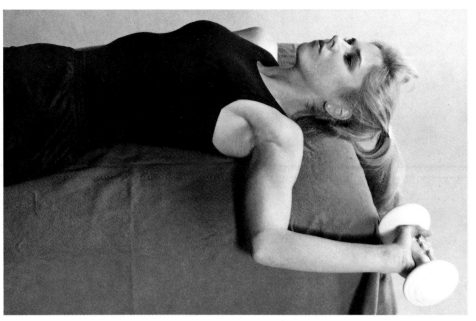

FIGURE 11-16. Anterior capsule stretch: Shoulder.

The Intermediate Phase

The second major phase of a general shoulder rehabilitation program commences when the patient has attained flexibility of at least 90 degrees abduction and 90 degrees flexion. The increase in the functional range of motion allows a more aggressive approach to stretching of the joint capsule and surrounding musculature. Instruct the patient on how to hold the shoulder at the end of range for 10 seconds with a 5-second rest between consecutive stretches. Also, increase the number of repetitions from 10 to 15 and have the patient stretch the shoulder move vigorously with each repetition. For warmup, use the saw, cross-body saw, and the pendulum exercises.

Stretching Exercises

Expand the wand exercises to include shoulder extension. To do this, have the patient stand and grasp the stick with both hands behind the body (Fig. 11-15). While he keeps his elbows straight, have him move the stick backwards away from the body as far as possible. Then, with the stick in front of the abdomen, have him perform exercises of horizontal abduction/adduction. Now, with the wand elevated to shoulder height, have him move the stick with the elbows extended toward the midline for adduction and away from the midline for abduction.

Anterior Capsule Stretches. Two exercises are used to stretch the anterior capsule. The first, which is performed supine on a table with the involved shoulder over the edge, involves bending the elbow 90 degrees as a 2-pound weight is placed in the hand (Fig. 11-16). The patient should let the weight pull the shoulder into some extension and maximal external rotation. The second stretch, which is performed standing, facing a corner of the wall with the shoulder abducted and each elbow flexed to 90 degrees (Fig. 11-17). The patient places the ulnar side of the forearm against a right-angled wall and then moves the torso forward. This motion causes the shoulder to abduct horizontally to the end of range. As an exercise to stretch the anterior/inferior

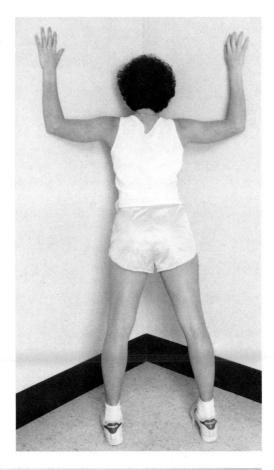

FIGURE 11-17. Anterior capsule stretch: Shoulder.

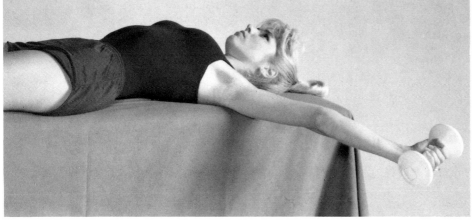

FIGURE 11-18. Anterior inferior capsule stretch: Shoulder.

capsule, have the patient supine with the shoulder over the table edge in a position of 135 degrees of abduction. Place a 2-pound weight in the hand. This will cause the shoulder to move into horizontal abduction (Fig. 11-18).

Inferior Capsule Stretches.   Two other exercises can be used to stretch the inferior capsule. In the first, the patient is again in the supine position on a table with the shoulder over the edge and in full flexion (Fig. 11-19). Have the patient grasp a 2-pound weight in the hand to cause the shoulder to stretch into fuller flexion. In the second, have the patient stand and reach overhead with a 2-pound weight while gently pushing the upper arm with the opposite hand in order to move the weighted limb into maximal abduction (Fig. 11-20).

71

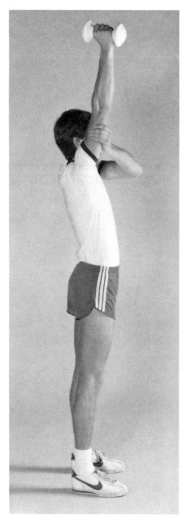

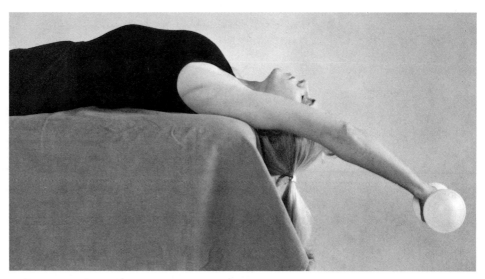

FIGURE 11-19.   Inferior capsule stretch: Shoulder.

FIGURE 11-20.   Inferior capsule stretch: Shoulder.

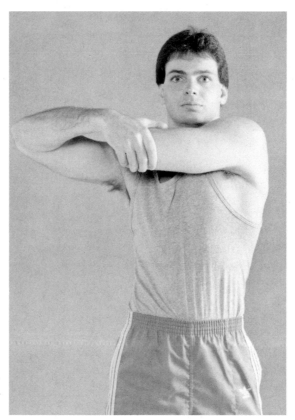

FIGURE 11-21.   Posterior capsule stretch: Shoulder.

Posterior Capsule Stretches.   The posterior capsule can be stretched by holding the involved arm in horizontal adduction and by placing the hand near the opposite shoulder (Fig. 11-21). The patient then gently pulls the arm across the body by using the hand of the uninvolved shoulder placed just above the elbow.

Progressive Resistance Exercises

At this stage, initiate resistance exercises of the shoulder and elbow to strengthen the upper musculature. Because the long heads of the triceps and biceps brachii muscles are active during motion at two joints, it is important to include elbow exercises with shoulder injury. Start resistance exercises with one set of 10 repetitions and progress to three sets of 10 repetitions. A 1-minute rest period occurs between each set. The patient may start with resistance using rubber tubing (e.g., surgical tubing, Theraband) secured on a stable object. The patient may later advance to using free weights (i.e., 2 pounds) as tolerated.

All exercises should be performed with little or no shoulder joint pain. Complaints of muscular fatigue and discomfort usually do not warrant cessation of the exercise and are usually an exercise goal. Often, the patient complains of pain only during certain parts of the range of motion (e.g., painful arc), and exercises should be modified to avoid this painful range. During abduction and flexion, the painful arc usually occurs at mid-range when the greater tuberosity glides under the coracoacromial arch.[9]

Shoulder Flexion Exercises. Shoulder flexion may be performed in either the sitting or the standing position. The patient executes this exercise with the elbows straight, the shoulder in neutral rotation, and the forearm in neutral pronation/supination (i.e., thumb up position). Have the patient place the hand of the involved shoulder in the loop of the rubberband, move the shoulder into flexion, and attempt to pull the band apart. The contraction should be held for 5 seconds and then relaxed for 3 seconds. The patient will use the free weight with the same elbow and forearm positions, but only the injured shoulder is exercised (Fig. 11-22). This exercise works the coracobrachialis, the short head of biceps brachii, and the anterior deltoid muscles.

Shoulder Abduction Exercises. In shoulder abduction, the patient is either sitting or standing with injured arm held out slightly in front of the body.

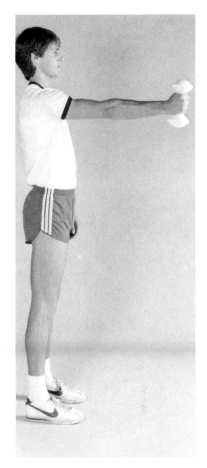

FIGURE 11-22. Flexion exercise: Shoulder.

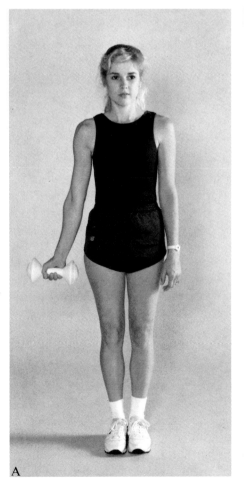
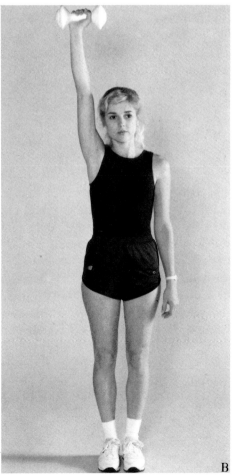

A   B

FIGURE 11-23A. Abduction exercise (starting position): Shoulder.

FIGURE 11-23B. Abduction exercise (ending position): Shoulder.

73

FIGURE 11-24A. Horizontal abduction exercise (starting position): Shoulder.

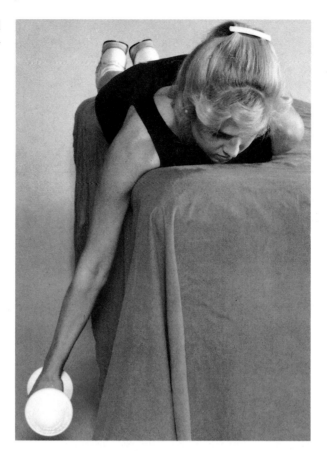

FIGURE 11-24B. Horizontal abduction exercise (ending position): Shoulder.

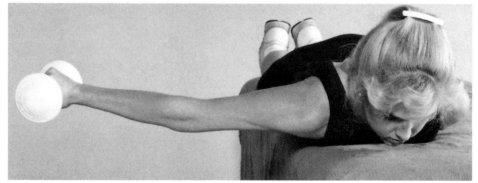

The hand is placed in the rubber tubing loop with the palm facing inward. The elbow is maintained in extension as the patient attempts to pull her hand up to the side. The contraction should be held for 2 to 5 seconds and then the patient returns to the starting position and rests for 3 seconds. When the patient is able to complete two sets of 10 repetitions with the rubber tubing, she may progress to free weights. Keeping the elbow straight and the hand to the side (Fig. 11-23A), the hand is raised upward and sideways over the head in the thumb-up position (Fig. 11-23B). This exercise strengthens the deltoid and supraspinatus muscles.

Horizontal Abduction Exercises. Horizontal abduction using rubber tubing is performed as the athlete either stands or sits. With the rubber tubing secured on a stable object, the hand is placed in the loop with the shoulder flexed to 90 degrees. While keeping the elbow straight he attempts to pull the rubber tubing apart and out to the side. To perform this exercise with free weights, have the athlete lie prone on a table and grasp the weight with the thumb up and start from a position in which the arm hangs down at the table side (Fig. 11-24A). While holding the weight in her hand, the athlete then abducts the arm 90 degrees (Fig. 11-24B). This exercise activates the posterior deltoid

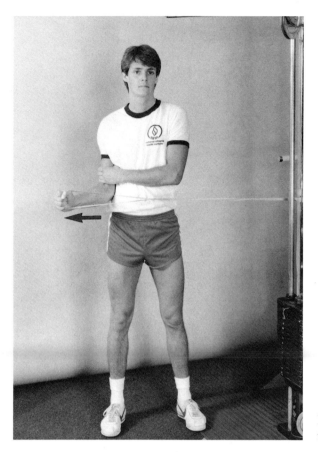

FIGURE 11-25. External rotation exercise: Shoulder.

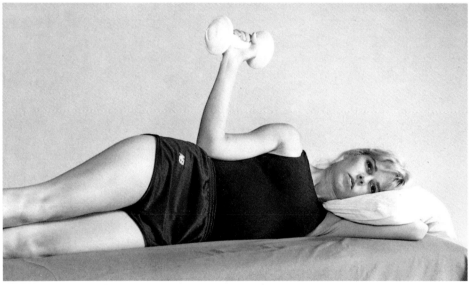

FIGURE 11-26. External rotation exercise: Shoulder.

rhomboids and the posterior rotator cuff muscles (the infraspinatus and the teres minor).

External Rotation Exercises. Next have the patient perform external rotation of the shoulder while standing. While holding the elbow close to the side and grasping it with his free hand to keep it in place, the patient flexes the arm to 90 degrees. Now, loop one end of the rubberband around a stationary object and slip his hand into the other end of the band (Fig. 11-25). Then, have him rotate the forearm externally against the resistance of the rubberband. Contract the muscle for 5 seconds, then relax it for 3 seconds.

When using free weights, the patient places herself in the lateral decubitus position with the injured side up (Fig. 11-26) and flexes the elbow to 90

75

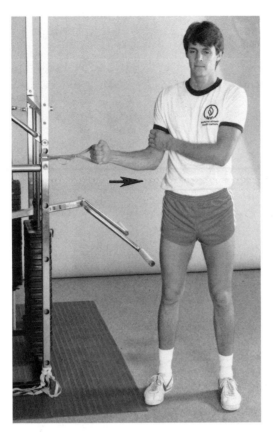

FIGURE 11-27. Internal rotation exercise: Shoulder.

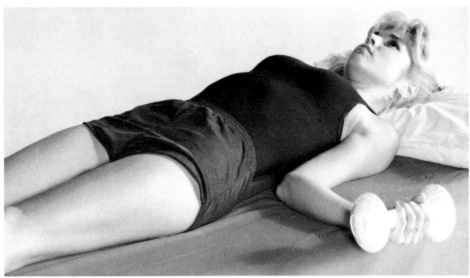

FIGURE 11-28. Internal rotation exercise: Shoulder.

degrees while stabilizing the upper arm at her side. Finally, have the patient grasp a 2-pound weight, hold the wrist in a neutral position, and rotate the forearm externally. This exercise strengthens the infraspinatus and teres minor muscles.

Internal Rotation Exercises. Internal rotation with rubberband resistance is also performed standing. The only difference is that the patient moves the forearm internally against the resistance of the rubberband (Fig. 11-27). When the patient is in the supine position on a table, have her work with a 2-pound free weight. She flexes the elbow to 90 degrees and holds it close to the body (Fig. 11-28) while rotating the forearm internally with the weight. This exercise will strengthen the subscapularis muscle.

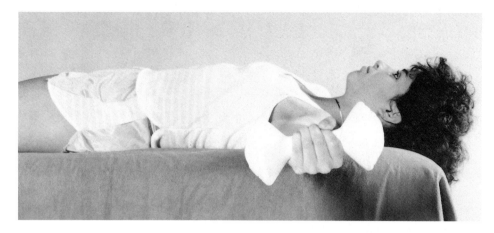

FIGURE 11-29A. Horizontal adduction exercise (starting position): Shoulder.

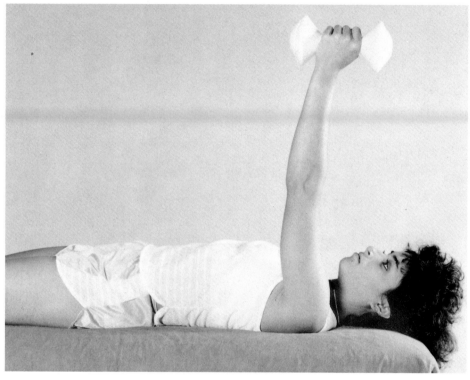

FIGURE 11-29B. Horizontal adduction exercise (ending position): Shoulder.

Horizontal Adduction Exercises. Horizontal adduction requires that the patient be supine on the table. Holding the elbow in extension and the shoulder in flexion to 90 degrees, the patient grasps a 2-pound weight in the thumb-up position (Fig. 11-29A). Starting from the neutral position, she moves the arm into maximum adduction (Fig. 11-29B). This exercise will strengthen the pectoralis major and the subscapularis muscles.

Shoulder Shrug Exercises. Have the patient perform shoulder shrugs while standing with a 2-pound weight in each hand. The scapulae are elevated and then depressed in a circular manner with scapular protraction and retraction (Fig. 11-7). This exercise will work the upper trapezius and levator scapulae muscles.

Shoulder Extension Exercises. Shoulder extension may be performed either with the patient lying prone on the table or in a standing position at the end of the table with the upper body flexed at the waist. The torso, now parallel to the floor, is supported by the uninvolved arm. The patient grasps a 2-pound weight and holds his elbow extended. He then moves the shoulder

77

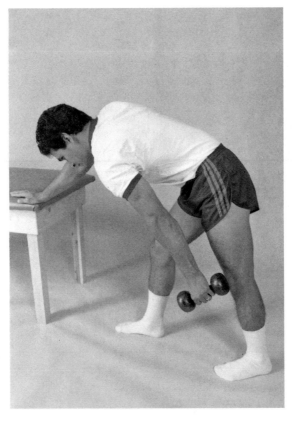
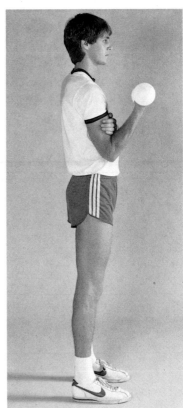

FIGURE 11-30. Extension exercise: Shoulder.

FIGURE 11-31. Flexion exercise: Elbow.

FIGURE 11-30   FIGURE 11-31

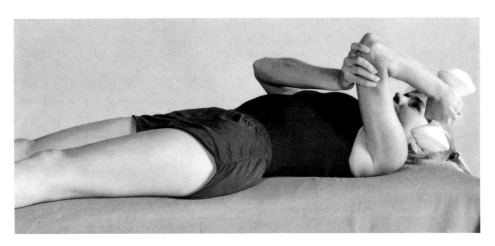

FIGURE 11-32. Extension exercise: Elbow.

into extension as tolerated (Fig. 11-30). The muscles targeted in this exercise are the latissimus dorsi, teres major and minor, and the infraspinatus.

Elbow Flexion and Extension Exercises. For elbow flexion, the patient is in a standing position as he grasps a 2-pound weight in the palm-up position (Fig. 11-31). Have the patient start the exercise in maximum elbow extension and move the forearm into as much flexion as can be tolerated. This maneuver will exercise the biceps brachii muscle.

For elbow extension, the patient is in the supine position on a table (Fig. 11-32) and uses free weights. Have her flex both the shoulder and the elbow to 90 degrees. While holding a 2-pound weight, and with the forearm in the neutral position, have the patient gradually extend the forearm at the elbow. This will work the triceps brachii.

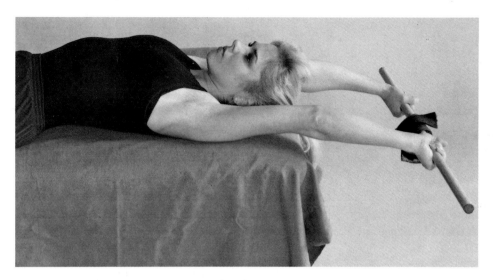

FIGURE 11-33. Wand flexion stretch: Shoulder.

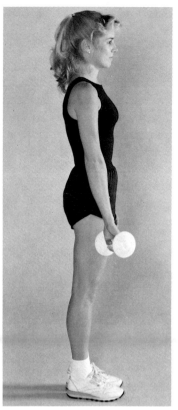

FIGURE 11-34A. Abduction exercise with internal rotation (Starting position): Shoulder.

Home Program

Instruct the patient in self-stretching of the rotator cuff and inferior capsule. Have him also perform the rubberband exercises with the same number of sets and repetitions as in therapy to increase endurance.

The Advanced Phase

This phase concentrates on the progressive return to normal function. In general, the patient continues the self-stretching exercises of the rotator cuff and inferior capsule as normal strength and endurance return to the musculature of the upper extremity. In this phase, the warmup period features pendulum exercises, which are performed as the patient holds a 2-pound weight to offer greater traction (Fig. 11-6). The same weight is also attached to a wand to achieve increased stretching during the wand exercises (e.g., Fig. 11-33).

Abduction with Internal Rotation Exercises

To the resistive exercises of this phase, add abduction with internal rotation exercises. The athlete stands with the arm at her side and rotates the shoulder internally to pronate the forearm (Fig. 11-34A). Then, moving the arm in a diagonal direction of abduction, she aims to achieve a goal of 90 degrees of abduction at 30 to 40 degrees in front of the coronal position (Fig. 11-34B). This position is used because it aligns the supraspinatus muscle parallel to the arm movement. In fact, the electromyographic output of the supraspinatus is greatest in this position.[7]

Continue to increase the free weights until the patient can safely transfer to the Nautilus machines for the resistance exercises. The athlete will usually reach this point when two sets of 10 repetitions can be executed while utilizing 10 pounds of free weights. It is best to have the athlete perform shoulder extension exercises on the Nautilus pullover unit because it mimics the shoulder extension that occurs in throwing, swimming, and racquet sports (Fig. 11-35). Other free-weight exercises used in the intermediate phase that may be advanced to Nautilus equipment are shoulder flexion (Fig. 11-36), horizontal abduction (Fig. 11-37), horizontal adduction (Fig. 11-38), elbow flexion (Fig. 11-39), and elbow extension (Fig. 11-40).

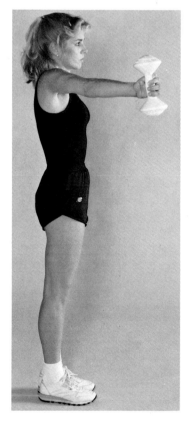

FIGURE 11-34B. Abduction exercise with internal rotation (ending position): Shoulder.

79

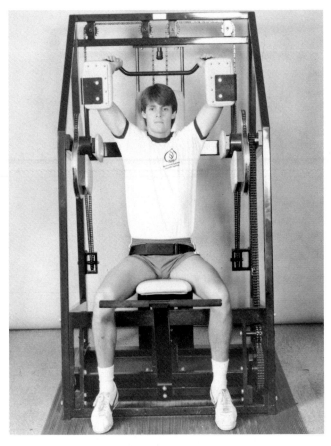

FIGURE 11-35. Extension exercise on Nautilus: Shoulder.

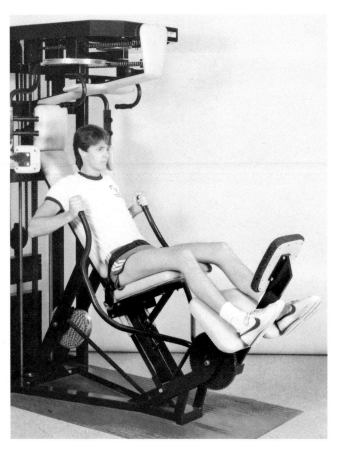

FIGURE 11-36. Flexion exercise on Nautilus: Shoulder.

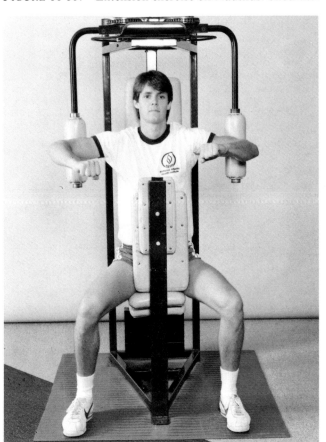

FIGURE 11-37. Horizontal abduction exercise on Nautilus: Shoulder.

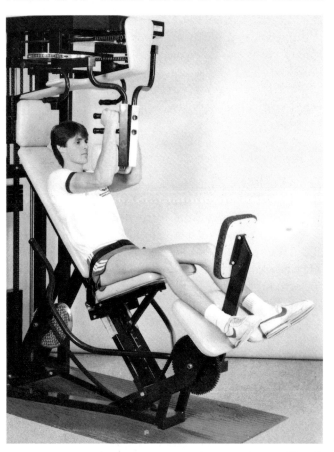

FIGURE 11-38. Horizontal adduction exercise on Nautilus: Shoulder.

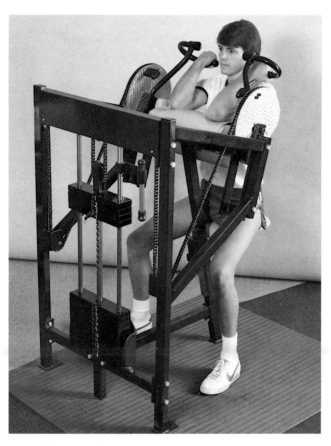

FIGURE 11-39.   Flexion exercise on Nautilus: Elbow.

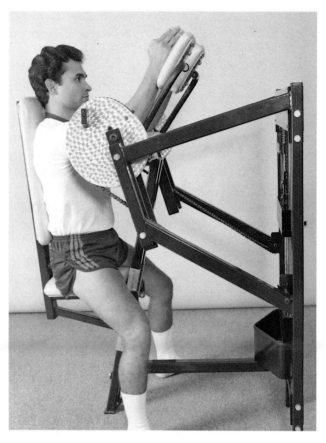

FIGURE 11-40.   Extension exercise on Nautilus: Elbow.

Throwing Program

Once the athlete's injured extremity has been cleared for throwing, he is ready to start the return to training. Now, before each throwing session, have him heat the joint for 15 minutes with hotpacks, whirlpool immersions, hot showers, and so on. The heat causes loosening of the connective tissue and increases the circulation.[4] After each throwing session, the joint should be iced for 10 to 15 minutes to decrease cellular damage and to lessen the body's natural inflammatory response to microtrauma.[11] Stretching exercises for the body in general, and for the elbow or shoulder in particular, should be performed though lightly, immediately after heating. They should also be repeated more vigorously immediately before icing.

The first 2 weeks of throwing are characterized by lobbing the ball on alternate days. The tosses not to exceed 30 feet. Throwing should be limited to two or three times per week and from 10 or 15 minutes per session. These throwing sessions are held on days when the regular strengthening program is not performed.[14]

The third week is characterized by increasing the throwing distance to 40 feet and the throwing time from 15 to 20 minutes per session. The intensity of throws (lobbing) and the frequency of sessions (2 to 3 times per week) remain unchanged.

The fourth week consists of increasing the throwing distance to 60 feet, allowing an occasional straight throw instead of the customary lobs (but only at one-half effort). Also, increase the throwing time per session from 20 to 25 minutes. The frequency of the sessions per week remains the same.

After the fourth week, place the athlete on a stepwise program of 9 days rather than 7; that is, sessions of throwing are held on 2 consecutive days followed by rest of 1 day, then throwing for 2 days, and so on. Progression from one step to the next (i.e., from lobbing to throwing) depends on the response of the shoulder or elbow to throwing, (i.e., whether or not there is pain or discomfort during throwing).

If there is no pain or discomfort during throwing, then allow progression to the next sequence of steps. Step 1 involves long, easy throws from the deepest portion of the outfield to home plate. They are throws in which the ball barely reaches home plate after numerous bounces. This type of throwing should be done for 25 to 30 minutes per session. Step 2 requires stronger throws from mid-outfield as the ball gets to home plate after five or six bounces. These sessions should last 30 minutes each. Step 3 focuses on throws that are short and crisp and have a relatively straight trajectory from the short outfield as they make their way back to home plate in one bounce. The length of the sessions is the same as that for Step 2.

Next, at Step 4, the athlete reaches what is a great step psychologically. At this step he begins returning to throwing at his normal position as shortstop, pitcher, catcher, and so on. The throws should be at one-half to three-quarter speed and emphasis should be placed on technique and accuracy. Step 5 is the same as Step 4 except that the effort of throwing should equal three-fourths to seven-eights of a maximal effort. Step 6 is different only in that throws are now at 100 percent of effort. Step 7, the final step, is the return to game competition.

Special Rehabilitation Protocols: The Shoulder

Impingement Syndrome

The major difference that characterizes "special" conditions over the "basic" ones discussed above for the shoulder is the severity of the weakness and the lack of mobility that the patient presents with as a result of surgery and subsequent immobilization.[3,16,17] The patient with a resection of the coracoacromial ligament can pass through the phases in a rapid manner.

Mobilization is initiated to restore physiological and accessory motion. In particular, we emphasize caudal glides of the humeral head in the glenoid to increase the available space between the acromion and the humerus.[5] In addition to exercises for stretching, add exercises for internal rotation, external rotation, and abduction with internal rotation. A strong rotator cuff is necessary to depress the humeral head in the glenoid during overhead activities.[8]

It is important to attain a strong rotator cuff through the rotator cuff exercises *before* initiating shoulder flexion and abduction (i.e., overhead) exercises. If shoulder flexion and abduction exercises are started prematurely, the result will be a return to the original pathokinesis (i.e., a drifting of the humeral head superiorly against the acromion).

In addition to strengthening the rotator cuff prior to starting abduction and flexion exercises, impingement may be avoided by having the patient perform these exercises only to 90 degrees of flexion and abduction. Increase the range of exercise movements periodically, but never allow the impingement of pain.

Two exercises that are important in the prevention of impingement are shoulder shrugs and push-ups. Shrugs help to strengthen the upper trapezius. The trapezius functions to upwardly rotate the scapula, thus allowing the acromion to elevate and not to contact the rotator cuff and biceps tendon. Push-ups with the arms abducted to 90 degrees will strengthen the serratus anterior. The inferior portion of this muscle can act independently from the superior portion to upwardly rotate the scapula.

Rotator Cuff

Rehabilitation following surgical repair of rupture of the rotator cuff is lengthy and characterized by slow progress. It requires an average of 12 to 14 months for an athlete to return to a level of activity that was maintained prior to injury.[6] Following surgery, the arm is placed in a sling or abduction splint for 2 to 4 weeks. After immobilization, the first month of rehabilitation consists of passive range of motion exercises necessary to restore range of motion. This is followed by therapy consisting of passive range of motion exercises as well as active and assisted range of motion exercises. Active and assisted range of motion exercises includes wand exercises and wall-slide exercises. General mobilization to restore accessory motion may also be utilized.

After 2 months of rehabilitation, the patient should have close to full range of passive motion of the shoulder. During the next month, have the patient continue stretching the shoulder and strengthening the rotator cuff by abduction. Also be sure that exercises of internal rotation and horizontal abduction are emphasized.

After 3 months of rehabilitation, the patient should be exercising the other shoulder muscles to increase overall strength (e.g., extension, horizontal adduction, etc.), while still performing stretching exercises. The stretching may now include advanced capsule stretching of the posterior, anterior, and inferior capsule.

At 7 months, Cybex isokinetic evaluation of the shoulder musculature is performed. We test shoulder flexion/extension, abduction/adduction, and internal/external rotation. Slow speed (60°/sec) and fast speed (300°/sec) testing is performed for flexion/extension and abduction/adduction. But only fast-speed testing is performed for internal/external rotation because slow-speed testing may trigger inflammation of the rotator cuff. The results of these tests are used to analyze specific weakness of muscle groups in order to assure that proper exercise to decrease these weaknesses are performed prior to beginning a return to the skills of a sport.

By now, the patient has begun performing general shoulder strengthening exercises on an exercise machine (e.g., Nautilus, Universal). The goal for return to the skills of a sport (e.g., throwing) is 8 months postsurgery for most patients, although a great deal of variability from one patient to the next occurs. The program of specific rotator cuff strengthening, general shoulder strengthening, and capsular stretching continues as long as the patient uses the shoulder to any great degree in activities of daily living and sports.

Anterior Reconstruction

The modified Bristow reconstruction and anterior staple capsulorrhaphy surgeries are used to correct anterior instability of the glenohumeral joint. Postsurgically, strict immobility of the shoulder must be maintained for 3 to 4 weeks. As a result, the patient often presents with marked range of motion losses. These may be equal to zero degrees of external rotation and more than 90 degrees of flexion/abduction. These losses are even greater if the Bristow reconstruction itself is performed.

The most difficult range of motion to regain is the range of external rotation motion. Initially, a goal of approximately 80 degrees of external rotation is adequate.[12,18] Have the patient start with immediate gentle stretching while shoulder internal/external rotation is in neutral. Then proceed to saw exercises.

83

This entire group of exercises should all be performed three to four times a day at the rehabilitation center and 10 times a day at home. The next step is aggressive mobilization, which should include caudal and posterior accessory glides as well as physiological flexion and abduction stretches. Assess the ranges of active and passive motion weekly; do not initiate physiological external rotation stretching unless there is little progress after 3 to 4 weeks of therapy.

Ninety degrees of abduction and of flexion should be obtained after 2 to 3 weeks of therapy. Once these criteria are met, start general shoulder strengthening exercises. More importantly, in order to offer dynamic stability to an anterior reconstruction or stapling at this point in the rehabilitation program, be sure to emphasize exercises that strengthen the anterior shoulder musculature, especially the subscapularis.[20] These strengthening exercises include internal rotation from the neutral position to full internal rotation, shoulder flexion, and horizontal adduction from 70 degrees of horizontal abduction to neutral. When a satisfactory range of motion is obtained and when the strength of the shoulder flexors, internal rotators, and horizontal adductors approaches approximately 50 percent of normal, then initiate exercises to strengthen the musculature of the noninvolved shoulder. This program should conclude with work on the Nautilus prior to any return to the athlete's sport.

Posterior Reconstruction

The goal of posterior reconstruction of the shoulder is to limit posterior shoulder instability. Rehabilitation after surgery for posterior reconstruction mimics rehabilitation after surgery for anterior reconstruction. Exercises in both programs are performed to limit the range of motion with the intent of offering dynamic stability to the reconstructed side of the joint. For posterior reconstruction, this includes external rotation, horizontal abduction from the neutral position to full horizontal abduction, and shoulder extension from the 70-degree flexion position to full extension. Contraindications after surgery are mobilizations that include anterior/posterior glides and forced horizontal adduction and/or internal rotation. These mobilizations are avoided because of the undue stress they place on the posterior capsule. Aggressive stretching of the anterior capsule is, however, important because it allows adequate anterior humeral glide and thus decreases any force on the posterior capsule.

Basic Rehabilitation Protocol—The Elbow

The Starting Phase

Like the rehabilitation of the shoulder after surgery, that of the elbow after surgery has the same major aims: to restore the range of motion and to decrease pain. A flexible joint requires less energy to move and can move further in its range.[10,15] Unfortunately, the most common complication after elbow injury is elbow stiffness.[19] Elbow stiffness results from bony incongruity, degenerative changes of the articular surfaces, and/or inelasticity of the surrounding soft tissue. Physical therapy is directed at correction of the latter mechanism of joint stiffness.

During the starting phase, physiological stretching is useful in decreasing elbow pain and increasing the range of motion. At this time, have the patient perform Grade I and II physiological stretching (Fig. 11-12). This includes elbow flexion/extension and forearm pronation/supination.[13] Passive motion is also useful because it helps the patient become less apprehensive about

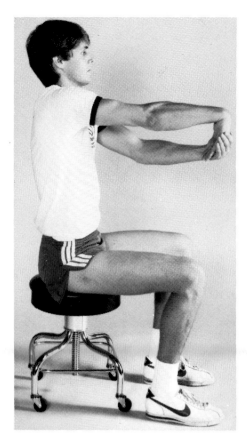 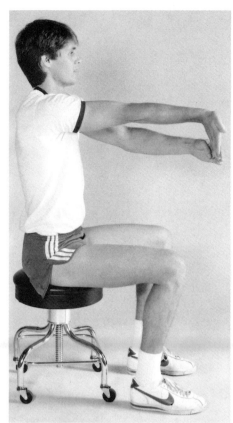

FIGURE 11-41. Extension stretch: Wrist.   FIGURE 11-42. Flexion stretch: Wrist.

moving the elbow into ranges that were prohibited during the immobilization stage.

In addition to stretching at the elbow, stretches of the musculature that originate at the elbow may be initiated in the starting phase. To accomplish this, have the patient stretch the common flexor and common extensor masses with exercises for wrist extension (Fig. 11-41) and for wrist flexion (Fig. 11-42), respectively. These and other self stretches mentioned below should be held in the stretch position for 5 to 10 seconds and should be repeated from 5 to 15 times per session each day.

The Intermediate Phase

Strengthening exercises may be initiated at the elbow as early as 1 week after the stretching program is initiated. Exercises for the elbow rehabilitation are performed at the elbow, forearm, wrist and hand. (Flexion and extension exercises at the elbow are included in the section on shoulder rehabilitation exercises.) Elbow rehabilitation exercises should be performed in one to three sets of 5 to 20 repetitions.

Strengthening Exercises

Finger Flexion.   Finger flexion exercises may be performed using a tennis ball or Grafna Thera-Putty (Graham-Field, New Hyde Park, New York). Repetitive squeezes of either object strengthens the flexor mass and improves grip strength necessary for throwing and racquet sports. The specific elbow

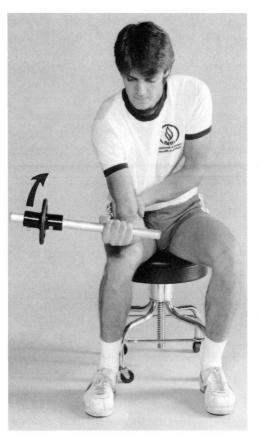

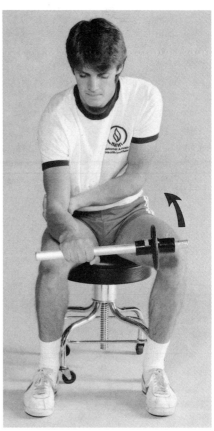

FIGURE 11-43. Pronation exercise: Forearm.

FIGURE 11-44. Supination exercise: Forearm.

muscles strengthened are the flexor digitorum superficialis, flexor digitorum profundus, and flexor pollicis longus.

Forearm Pronation. With the elbow flexed to 90 degrees, have the patient perform this exercise while sitting and using a weighted bar for resistance (Fig. 11-43). Resistance is offered by the bar from the complete palm-up position (full forearm supination) to neutral pronation/supination. These exercises strengthen the pronator teres and the pronator guadratus muscles. The pronator teres muscle crosses the elbow joint, and motion at the elbow occurs with forearm pronation and supination.

Forearm Supination. This exercise is similar to that for forearm pronation. It is performed from the fully pronated forearm position to the neutral pronation/supination position (Fig. 11-44). The muscles exercised in this movement are the biceps and the spinator.

Deviation. The *radial* deviation exercise is performed while sitting or standing. Have the patient start with a weighted bar in hand and pointed forward; then have him lift the bar, led by the thumb and using the wrist only (Fig. 11-45). This exercise strengthens the muscles that radially deviate the wrist: the flexor carpi radialis and the extensor carpi radialis longus muscles. Both of these muscles cross the elbow joint. The *ulnar* deviation exercise is similar to that for radial deviation. Have the athlete move the weighted bar into ulnar deviation as tolerated. This exercise is used to strengthen the wrist ulna deviators: the flexor carpi ulnaris and the extensor carpi ulnaris.

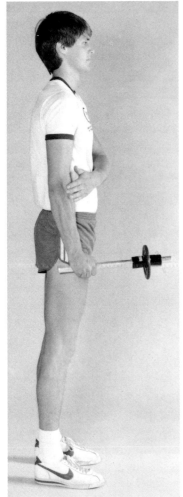

FIGURE 11-45. Radial deviation exercise: Wrist.

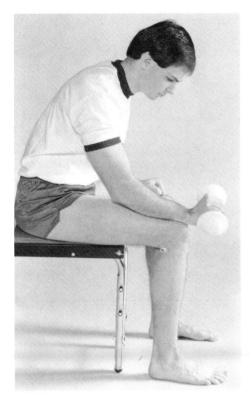 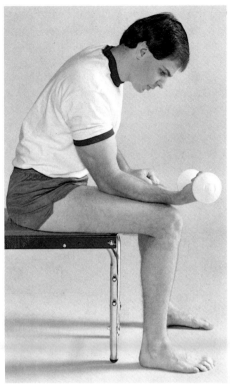

FIGURE 11-46. Extension exercise: FIGURE 11-47. Flexion exercise: Wrist.
Wrist.

Wrist Extension. The patient should perform this exercise while seated and keeping the forearm stabilized either on the thigh or a table. The weight should be held with the overhand grip and the forearm pronated (Fig. 11-46). The hand is lowered into a fully flexed position and then raised into extension. This exercise strengthens the wrist extensor group, that is, the extensor carpi radialis longus, the extensor carpi radialis brevis, and the extensor carpi ulnaris. All these muscles cross the elbow joint.

Wrist Flexion. This exercise is similar to the wrist extension exercise except that the weight is gripped with an underhand position (Fig. 11-47). The weight is lowered into a fully flexed position and then raised up into extension. This exercise strengthens the flexor muscles of the wrist, that is, the flexor carpi ulnaris, the flexor carpi radialis, and the palmaris longus. Stretching during the intermediate phase is more aggressive than it is in the starting phase.

Stretching Exercises

If the patient has not regained full range of motion, stretching is more aggressive during this intermediate phase than the starting phase. Physiological stretches are continued to attain complete elbow flexion/extension and forearm pronation/supination range. Grade I and II physiological stretches are used during the starting phase, but during this intermediate phase Grade III and IV (Fig. 11-12) stretches to the end of range are used. Accessory mobilization may also be inititiated using caudal glides of the ulna on the humerus and anterior/posterior, as well as posterior/anterior glides of the head of the radius on the ulna.[13]

Elbow Extension Stretch. This exercise is accomplished best with the patient

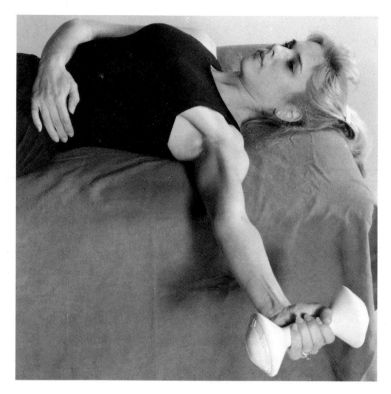

FIGURE 11-48.   Extension stretch: Elbow.

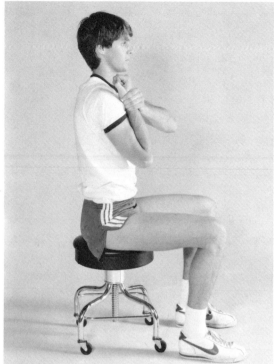

FIGURE 11-49.   Flexion stretch: Elbow.

supine and a 2-pound weight attached to the wrist or hand, thus increasing the force being exerted for extension (Fig. 11-48).

Forearm Pronation/Supination Stretch.   The patient performs this stretching exercise by using a weighted bar in the same starting position as that used in the wrist pronation/supination strengthening exercise (Fig. 11-43).

Elbow Flexion Stretch.   This exercise is done with the use of the other arm to give force for greater stretch. When performed seated as depicted in Figure 11-49, this exercise stretches the triceps muscle and increases the flexion of motion at the elbow.

The Advanced Phase

During the advanced phase, wrist and elbow flexion and extension strengthening exercises may be performed on an exercise machine (e.g., Nautilus, Universal). Exercises utilizing free weights should be continued to strengthen muscles controlling pronation/supination and radial/ulnar deviation. In addition, an exercise program for the shoulder, as previously described, should be initiated.

Also, during the early part of the advanced stage, initiate a total body-fitness program. This program may begin in the starting phase but does not become critical until the advanced stage. This program should consist of running, swimming, and/or bicycling to develop cardiovascular fitness and leg strength and endurance.[15] This is especially important for athletes who engage in sports that use predominantly the musculature of the upper extremity (e.g., tennis, baseball, racquetball) but also require strong lower extremity musculature.

Once the range of elbow motion is reestablished within normal limits and in satisfactory strength, which is usually indicated when the athlete reaches plateaus at normal or near-normal resistance values, initiate the athlete's return to the skills of his or her sport. For guidelines in returning to throwing sports, please refer to the throwing protocol described in the shoulder rehabilitation section above.

References

1. Coonrad RW, Hooper WR: Tennis elbow: Its course, natural history, conservative and surgical management. *J Bone Jt Surg* 1973;55-A:1177–1182.
2. Cooper DL, Fair J: Contrast baths and pressure treatment for ankle sprains. *Phys Sports Med* 1979;7(4):143.
3. Crenshaw AH, Kilgore WE: Surgical treatment of bicipital tenosynovitis. *J Bone Jt Surg* 1966;48-A:1496–1502.
4. Greenberg RS: The effects of hot packs and exercise on local blood flow. *Phys Ther* 1972;52:273–278.
5. Gould JA, Davis GH (eds): The shoulder, in *Orthopaedic and Sports Physical Therapy.* St Louis, Mosby, 1985 vol. 2, pp 497–517.
6. Jobe FW, Rotator cuff injuries in young people. Read before the Seventh Annual Meeting of the American Orthopaedic Society for Sports Medicine, Lake Tahoe, NV, June 1981.
7. Jobe FW, Moynes DR: Delineation of diagnostic criteria and a rehabilitation program for rotator cuff injuries. *Am J Sports Med* 1982;10:336–339.
8. Kent BE: Functional anatomy of the shoulder complex: A review. *Phys Ther* 1971;51:867–888.
9. Kessel L, Watson M: The painful arc syndrome: Clinical classifications as a guide to management. *J Bone Jt Surg* 1977; 59-B:166–172.
10. Klafs CE, Arnheim DD: *Modern Principles of Athletic Training* St. Louis, Mosby, 1977.
11. Knight, KL: Effect of hypothermia on immediate care of athletic injuries. *Ath Train* 1976;11:6–9.
12. Lombardo SJ, Kerlan RK, et al: The modified Bristow procedure for recurrent dislocation of the shoulder. *J Bone Jt Surg* 1976;58-A:256–261.
13. Maitland GD: *Peripheral Manipulation* ed 2. London, Butterworth's, 1977, pp 5–10.
14. Maitland GD: Treatment of the glenohumeral joint by passive movement. *Physiotherapy* 1983;69:3–7.
15. Morehouse L, Gross L: *Maximum Performance.* New York, Simon & Schuster, 1977.
16. Neer CS: Anterior acromioplasty for the chronic impingment syndrome in the shoulder. *J Bone Jt Surg* 1972;54-A:41–50.
17. Neer CS, Welsh RP: The shoulder in sports. *Orthop Clin* 1977;8:583–591.
18. Stoddard G: The physical rehabilitation of selected shoulder injuries. *Ath Train* 1978;13:34–39.
19. Tucker K: Some aspects of post-traumatic elbow stiffness. *Injury* 1978;9:216–220.
20. Turkel SJ, Panio MW, Marshall JL, Girgis FG: Stabilizing mechanisms preventing anterior dislocation of the glenohumeral joint. *J Bone Jt Surg* 1981;63-A:1208–1217.

Additional Reading

Aronen JG, Regan K: Decreasing the incidence of recurrance of first time anterior dislocations with rehabilitation. *Am J Sports Med* 1984,12:283–291.
Atwater AE: Biomechanics of overarm throwing movements and of throwing injuries. *Exerc Sport Sci Rev* 1979;7:43–85.
Moynes DR: Prevention of injury to the shoulder through exercise and therapy. *Clin Sports Med* 1983;2:413–422.
Neer CS: Impingement lesions. *Clin Orthop* 1983;173:70–77.

Pappas AM, Zawacki RM, McCarthy CF: Rehabilitation of the pitching shoulder. *Am J Sports Med* 1985;13:223–235.

Pappas AM, Zawacki RM, Sullivan TJ: Biomechanics of baseball pitching. A preliminary report. *Am J Sports Med* 1985;13:216–222.

Woods GW, Tullos HS, King JW: The throwing arm: Elbow joint injuries. *J Sports Med Suppl* 1973;1(4):43–47.

Zarins B, Rowe CR: Current concepts in the diagnosis and treatment of shoulder instability in athletes. *Med Sci Sports Exerc* 1984;15:444–448.

Knee

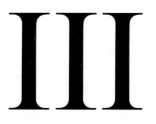

12 Arthroscopy

Lewis A. Yocum

General Considerations

Although the arthroscope only complements the normal physical examination of the joint, it is an instrument that allows the clinician to extend that examination to the joint's internal anatomy. The arthroscope also affords the surgeon an opportunity not only to identify pathology but often to correct it. An understanding of arthroscopy is thus essential to the sports orthopaedist.

Two points, however, must be stressed: arthroscopy is a skill that takes considerable time to master; arthroscopic findings only contribute to—and do not substitute for—a detailed history and physical examination of the patient's extremity. In addition, a necessary prerequisite before beginning arthroscopic evaluation of the knee is to check the range of motion of the hips, knees, and ankle. A thorough evaluation of the ligamentous stability of the joint is equally important. It should include both straight and rotatory as well as evaluation of patellar-tracking characteristics.

Surgical Procedure and Techniques

Once you are satisfied that you understand the gross anatomy and stability of the leg, begin the arthroscopy. Place the patient in a supine position on the operating table and institute effective general anesthesia. Local or regional anesthesia are viable options. In our experience, we have found that general anesthesia affords us the opportunity for a thorough ligamentous examination as well as a complete arthroscopic evaluation in a relaxed atmosphere from which very few complications arise. Once the patient is anesthetized, repeat the ligamentous examination and compare both extremities.

Next, apply a pneumatic cuff to the thigh and have it ready for use. Although controversy exists about using or not using a pneumatic cuff, a bloodless field does afford the surgeon a clearer visualization of the joint. Because most procedures are of relatively short duration, the complications are minimal. When a hemostatic cuff is used, apply an Esmarch bandage to exsanguinate the extremity before inflation. Generally, inflate the hemostatic cuff to a level of 100 mm Hg above systolic pressure. Then, sterily prep the lower extremity and drape it so that the leg is entirely free. Use a sterile stockinette over the extremity to allow free access to the knee.

The use of leg holder is essential. The holder can range from a simple lateral post to a more complex circumferential band, which will provide medio-lateral support as well as control rotation. The circumferential cuff often provides a venous tourniquet, and the surgeon should be aware of this. It may also prevent a figure-of-four position for a lateral compartment exploration.

Inject a total of 10 to 15 cc of bupivacaine (0.25%) with epinephrine (1:200,000) at the point of all proposed portals. Flex the knee to 90 degrees by holding the foot flat on the operating table. Usually, surgeons use an anterolateral portal first for insertion of the arthroscope. Next, carry out palpation of the patellar tendon, lateral tibial plateau, and femoral condyle. For the incision, select a point 1 cm above the lateral tibial plateau and about 1 cm lateral to the patellar tendon.

After an injection of anesthetic, make a stab wound with a #11 knife blade and carry the wound through the skin and subcutaneous tissue to the level of the capsule. Careful entry to the capsule is possible with a #11 blade, but further penetration should be avoided. This eliminates the need for a sharp trocar. If necessary, insert a small hemostat to enlarge the capsule and skin incisions. At all times, take care to prevent injury to articular surfaces.

Extend the limb and insert the hemostat carefully into the suprapatellar pouch in order to allow further dilation. Then, remove the clamp and return the knee to a 90-degree flexed posture. Next, insert the arthroscopic cannula with a blunt trocar in place and direct the cannula toward the intracondylar space. Once entry is made, bring the knee gently into extension and direct the cannula into a suprapatellar pouch. Withdraw the trocar and insert the arthroscope (Fig. 12-1). (We generally use a 4-mm 30-degree arthroscope.) Drape a small handheld camera sterilely and attach it to the end of the arthroscope in order to facilitate viewing.

Connect a 3-liter bag of saline through sterile tubing to the scope inflow in order to distend the joint slightly from the inflow. (Between 60 and 100 cc of fluid is generally required for adequate distention.) At this time, insert an egress cannula through a stab wound in the superomedial aspect of the knee. Make the stab wound approximately 1 cm medial to the patella, and 1 cm below the superior pole of the patella. Again, direct the cannula into the suprapatellar pouch, to avoid chondral damage (Fig. 12-1). Connect the egress to low continuous suction.

Inspection of the joint can now begin. Flex the foot of the table to allow free-ranging motion of the knee. Either sit or stand, but be certain to maintain sterile technique. (We prefer standing with the assistant holding the lower leg and adjusting the position according to the needs of the surgeon.)

Inspection must be systematic and thorough. First, inspect the suprapatellar pouch and patellofemoral joint (Fig. 12-2). Next, inspect the medial gutter as the scope is brought into the medial compartment. On entering the medial compartment, flex the knee to 30 to 40 degrees and apply a valgus stress. The scope is now in position between the femur and tibia and allows you to look directly at the medial meniscus (Fig. 12-3).

At this point, create an anteromedial portal by using a #11 blade. The use of a 21-gauge spinal needle aids in the selection of appropriate portal. Generally, a portal is selected 1 cm above the medial tibial plateau and 0.5 to 1 cm medial to the patellar tendon. Enlarge the portal with a hemostat; insert a nerve hook to prove the meniscus and to assist in examining the joint. Insert the arthroscope through the intercondylar space medial to the cruciate ligaments so that the posterior horn of the meniscus can be seen (Fig. 12-4).

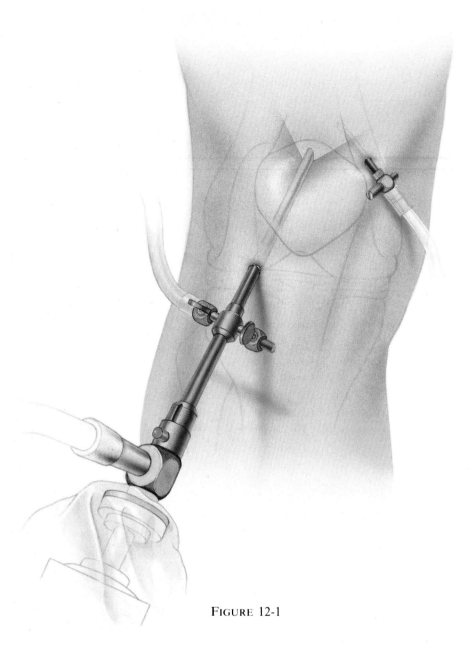

FIGURE 12-1

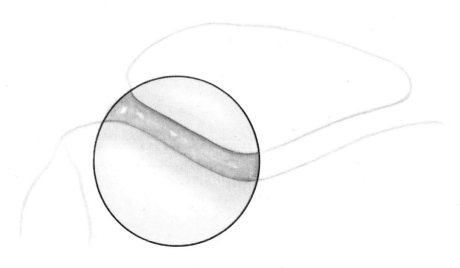

FIGURE 12-2.   Patellofemoral joint.

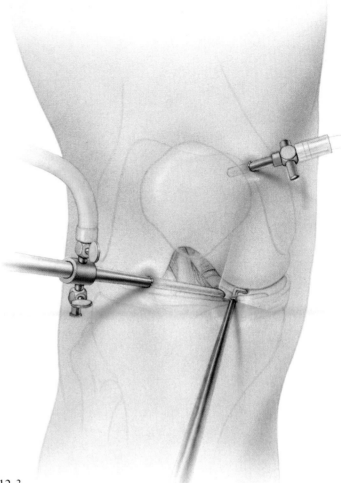

FIGURE 12-3

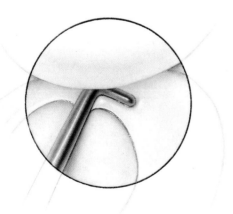

FIGURE 12-4. View of posterior horn medial meniscus.

This posterior inspection can be done through a transpatellar tendon approach as well, though we have found it rarely necessary to use this approach. If you decide to use this approach, select a portal 1 cm distal to the inferior tip of the patella in the midline. To facilitate the viewing of the entire medial compartment, use both a 30-degree as well as 70-degree arthroscope. The 70-degree arthroscope is beneficial for viewing posteriorly through the intracondylar space.

95

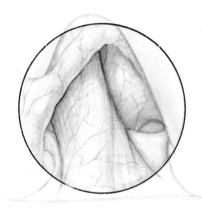

FIGURE 12-5. Transpatellar view of cruciate ligaments.

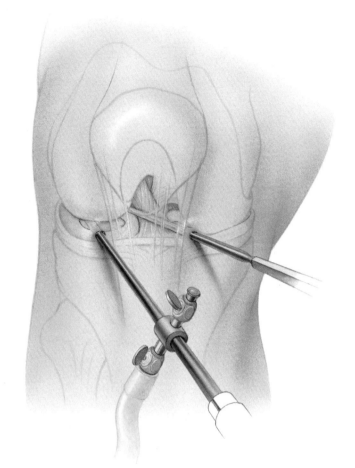

FIGURE 12-6

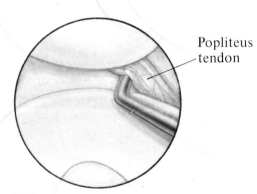

Popliteus tendon

FIGURE 12-7

Also inspect the intracondylar space by visualizing the cruciates (Fig. 12-5). Direct visualization of the cruciates during stress testing for anterior or posterior drawer can also be beneficial. Then, further flex the knee to 80 or 90 degrees, and rotate the hip externally to create a figure-of-four position. This produces varus stress and opens the lateral compartment for inspection (Fig. 12-6). Carry on an inspection of the entire lateral meniscus and popliteal tendon. Then, bring the knee back to a position of 30 to 40 degrees of flexion. Finally, inspect the lateral gutter and pay particular attention to the popliteal hiatus (Fig. 12-7).

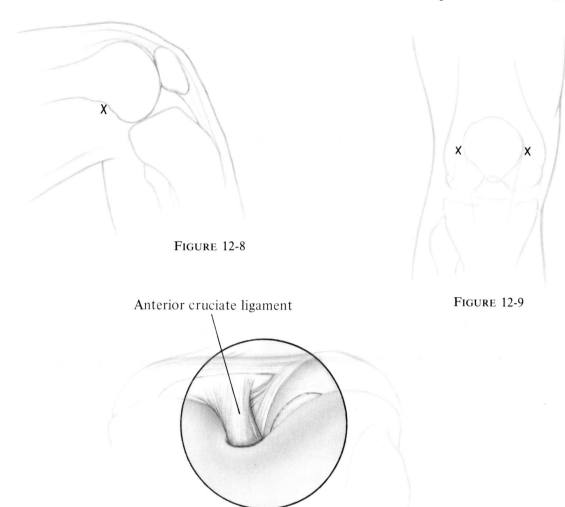

FIGURE 12-8

FIGURE 12-9

Anterior cruciate ligament

FIGURE 12-10

In most cases, the standard anterolateral and anteromedial portals are all that are necessary for adequate examination of the joint. Occasionally, a transpatellar tendon approach may be necessary. However, the arthroscopist should be thoroughly familiar with all portals to the joint.

A posteromedial approach (Fig. 12-8) is facilitated by distending the joint with saline and by flexing the knee to 90 degrees as the outflow is shut off. Next, rotate the leg externally. In the posteromedial corner of the knee, note the synovial bulge, which is located just posterior to the medial collateral ligament in the "soft spot." Inject local anesthetic over the proposed portal. On occasion, you can transilluminate the intracondylar space with the arthroscope by coursing it posteriorly in the knee. In this way, you can delineate neural structures that should be avoided. Entry into the posteromedial portal is facilitated again by using a 21-gauge spinal needle, by visualizing the anteromedial portal, and by determining the position necessary for entry into the posteromedial compartment. When satisfactory position is obtained, make a small stab wound with a #11 blade and insert the arthroscope into the posteromedial compartment.

Both on the medial and on the lateral aspects of the knee a midpatellar portal affords excellent visualization of the joint, especially at the anterior meniscal attachments (Fig. 12-9). Select a point just to the side of the patella. Then, bring the knee into 20 to 30 degrees of flexion. This range of flexion provides the best visualization of the anterior aspect of the joint (Fig. 12-10).

The portals we have described here afford the operating surgeon the best opportunities to evaluate the knee thoroughly.

References

1. Shahriaree H, *Ed. O'Connor's Textbook of Arthroscopic Surgery.* Philadelphia, Lippincott, 1984, pp 43–72.
2. Johnson LL: *Diagnostic and Surgical Arthroscopy: The Knee and Other Joints.* St. Louis, Mosby, 1981, pp 215–239.

Additional Reading

Eriksson E, Sebik A: Arthroscopy and arthroscopic surgery in a gas versus fluid medium. *Orthop Clin North Am* 1982;Apr 13:293–298.

McGinty JB: Arthroscopic removal of loose bodies. *Orthop Clin North Am* 1982;13: 313–328.

Mital MA, Karlin LI: Diagnostic arthroscopy in sports injuries. *Orthop Clin North Am* 1980;11:771–785.

Patellar Malalignment Syndromes

13

Clarence L. Shields, Jr.

General Considerations

Patients with patellar-tracking abnormalities will present with a variety of clinical syndromes. Mild cases will have aching pain on the anterior aspect of the knee. This discomfort will be aggravated by athletic activity and also by ascending and descending stairs. For some patients, the knee will actually give way and be followed by swelling and a feeling of insecurity in all twisting activities. Other patients will present with frequent dislocations while performing activities of daily living such as descending stairs or dancing.

Because patellar malalignment is so varied, it is difficult to determine when surgical intervention is justified. Several studies have reported good results with nonoperative management.[1-3] Other studies indicate that surgery is required.[4,5] Our routine radiographic evaluation of the patella is based on the Merchant view.[6] A physical examination will document patellar tracking, Q-angle, apprehension sign, genu valgus, patellar pain, patellar crepitus, and femoral and tibial torsion.

After the acute episode subsides, start the patients on a vigorous therapy program with quadriceps emphasis. For athletic events, be sure that the patellar stabilizing supports are used. Patients who are unable to control their symptoms with this protocol are candidates for surgical intervention.

Computerized tomography is able to distinguish significant differences in patellar centralization, patellar tilt, femoral sulcus angle, and depth of the femoral sulcus.[5] This technique has been refined to allow evaluation of the patellofemoral joint in extension, in 20 degrees of flexion, and in 45 degrees of flexion.[7] Following this protocol, we are undertaking a prospective study that uses computed tomography scores to determine the preferred surgical procedure. We recommend lateral retinacular release when the patellar lateral displacement is between 4 to 8 mm and when there is a positive patellar tilt and a relaxed sulcus angle of less than 165 degrees. Add medial patellar reefing when the lateral displacement is greater than 8 mm and the sulcus angle is greater than 165 degrees. A severely unstable patella will also have a tibial tubercle transfer. These patients have the additional findings of a negative patellar tilt and a sulcus angle greater than 175 degrees.

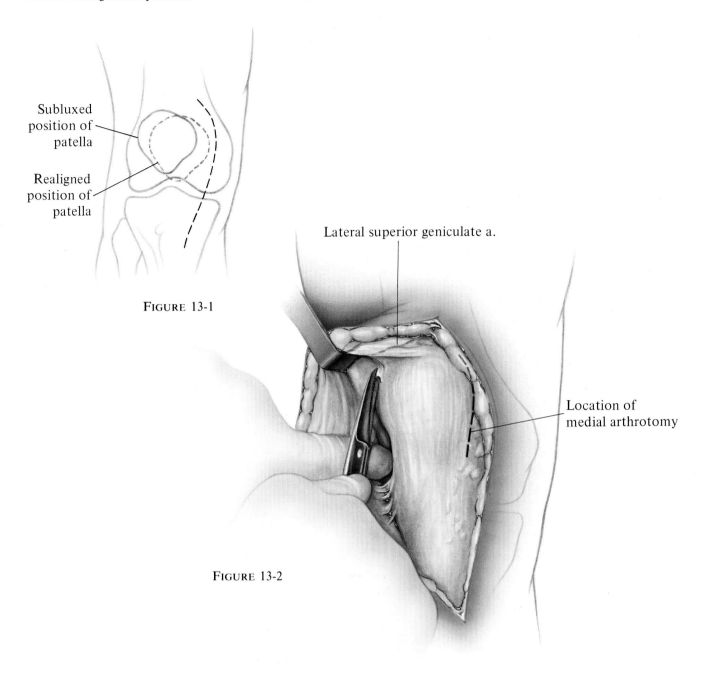

Subluxed
position of
patella

Realigned
position of
patella

FIGURE 13-1

Lateral superior geniculate a.

Location of
medial arthrotomy

FIGURE 13-2

Surgical Procedure and Techniques

Place the patient in the supine position on the operating table with a knee
bolster in position to allow 30 degrees of flexion. Wrap the extremity with
an Esmarch bandage for exsanguination and elevate the tourniquet to 250
mm of pressure. Utilize median parapatellar incision, but place it 1.5 cm
closer to the medial femoral epicondyle (Fig. 13-1). This is necessary since
the patella is further lateral than normal and the realigned position will place
the usual scar directly on top of the patella. The distal limb of the incision
extends to the level of the tibial tubercle only if it is going to be transferred.

Dissect the subcutaneous tissue laterally until the lateral patellar retinaculum
can be reached, and divide it with a knife until the synovium is visualized.
Develop the interval between the synovium and this layer with Mayo scissors.
Carry this interval proximally to the vastus lateralis muscle fibers, which
are usually 1.5 to 2 cm above the superior pole of the patella (Fig. 13-2).

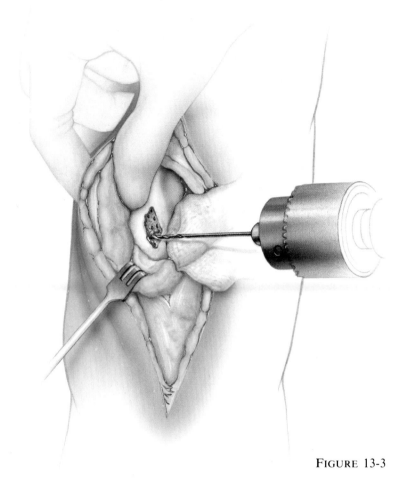

FIGURE 13-3

This may transect the lateral geniculate artery, which will be cauterized at tourniquet release. Sometimes it is necessary to open the synovium and release a thickened band of tissue attaching to the lateral border of the fat pad. In this case, carry the release distally along the lateral border of the patellar tendon.

Incise the medial patellar retinaculum with a knife. This capsular flap will include the vastus medialis muscle, which must be detached from the patella. Open the synovium and, along the same line, inspect the articular surface of the patellofemoral joint for chondromalacia. If shaving or drilling of the surface is required, place a wet saline-soaked sponge over the femoral groove to catch the debris (Fig. 13-3). Remove the gauze and irrigate the joint with Garamycin solution. In the patient requiring only a proximal realignment, initiate the medial side reefing.

In preparation for tibial tubercle transfer, outline the patellar tendon margins sharply with a knife prior to detaching the tubercle with an osteotome (Fig. 13-4). Dissect the tendon from the fat pad to allow free movement to the medial side. A periosteal flap is delineated with the same dimensions as the patellar tendon. The previous medial border of the tendon is now the lateral side of the flap, which you should now elevate with a distal base and roughen the exposed tibial cortex with a gouge (Fig. 13-5). The bone over the edge

101

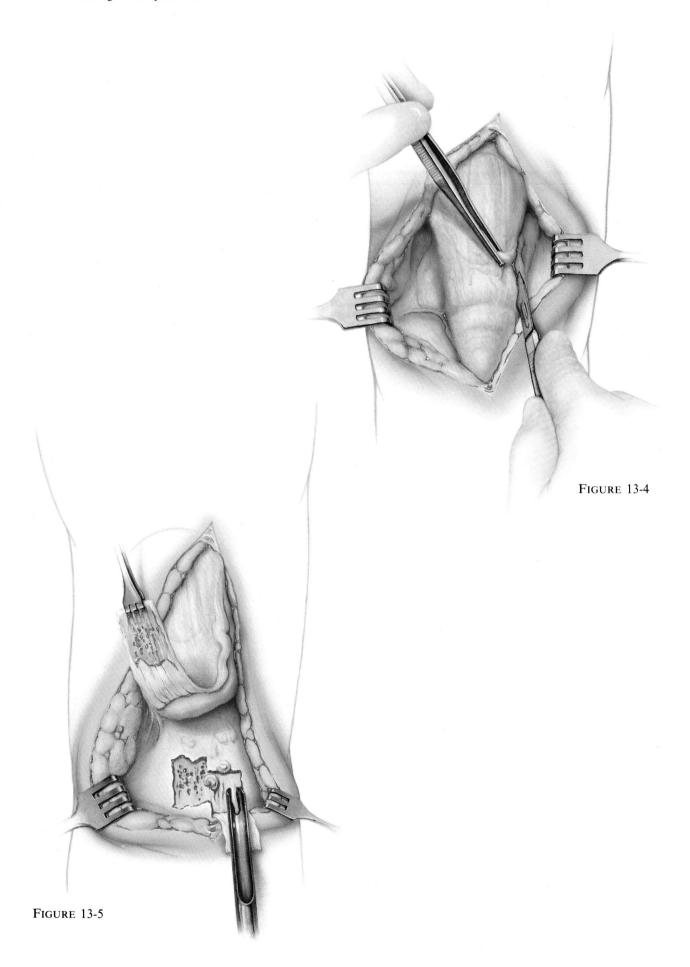

FIGURE 13-4

FIGURE 13-5

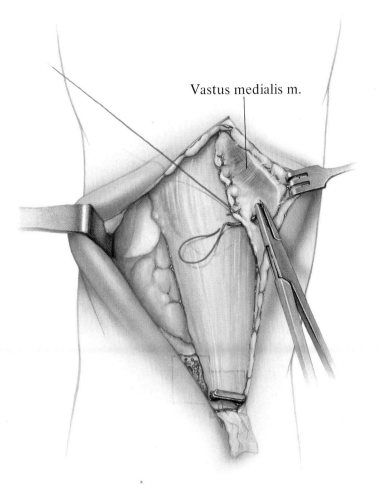

Vastus medialis m.

FIGURE 13-6

of the tibial tubercle may need trimming with ronguers in order to have the transfer lay flat on the tibia.

Choose the appropriate size of serrated staple and predrill the tibial cortex at the correct level. The goal is to transfer the extensor mechanism one tendon width medially (Fig. 13-5). If patella alta (high riding patella) is present, move the tendon 1 cm distally at the same time. Suture the periosteal flap over the transferred tendon with #1 Ethibond.

The proximal portion of the procedure is now completed. Close the synovium with a running #3–0 Dexon suture. Grasp the patella from the medial side with two towel clips and have the assistant hold them. Move the patella medially until 1.5 cm of the femoral groove is visible on the lateral patellar border. Now, suture the medial patellar retinaculum and the vastus medialis muscle on top of the patella with #1 Ethibond in a horizontal mattress fasion (Fig. 13-6). After placing four sutures, move the knee through 60 degrees of flexion and evaluate the patellar tracking. The patella must be centered and not advanced too far medially, especially in patients with a flat or shallow femoral groove. Occasionally, you will need to separate the vastus medialis muscle from the medial patellar retinaculum by a transverse cut at the lower border of the muscle. This will permit the medial reefing to be finely adjusted as needed for the proper patellar tracking. Complete the medial reefing only after inspecting the alignment. Leave the lateral retinaculum open.

Now, release the tourniquet and cauterize the lateral geniculate artery as required. Press a piece of thrombin-soaked Gelfoam into the bone at the original tendon insertion to control bleeding. Irrigate the wound with Garamycin solution and insert a ⅛-inch Reliavac drain under the lateral skin flap. Close the subcutaneous tissue with #3–0 Dexon and suture the skin with #4–0 clear nylon in subcuticular closure.

Postoperative Care and Rehabilitation

Immobilize the patient in molded splints, anteriorly and posteriorly, and allow him to ambulate with weightbearing as tolerated. Be sure that he does not perform quadriceps exercises. Remove the splints at 2 weeks and place the patient in a cylinder cast for 4 weeks. At 6 weeks in the postoperative period, strat the patient in physical therapy on the chondromalacia protocol (Chap. 23).

References

1. Crosby EB, Insall J: Recurrent dislocation of the patella. *J Bone Jt Surg* 1976;58-A:9–13.
2. Dehaven KE, Dolan WA, et al: chondromalacia patella in athletes. Clinical presentation and conservative management. *Am J Sports Med* 1979;7:5–11.
3. Henry JH, Crosland JW: conservative treatment of patellofemoral subluxation. *Am J Sports Med* 1979;7:12–14.
4. Cox, JS: Evaluation of Roux-Elmsie-Trillat procedure for knee extensor realignment. *Am J Sports Med* 1982;10:303–310.
5. Martinez S, Korobkin M, Fondren FB, et al: A device for computed tomography of the patellofemoral joint. *Am J Roentgenol* 1983;140:400–401.
6. Merchant AC, Mercer RL, Jacobsen RH, et al: Roentgenographic analysis of patello-femoral congruence. *J Bone Jt Surg* 1974;56-A:1391–1396.
7. Fondren FB, Kerlan RK, Shields CL, et al: Dislocation, subluxation and patellofemoral pain syndromes evaluated by computerized tomography. *J Bone Jt Surg.* Submitted for publication.
8. Fondren FB, Goldner JL, Bassett III FH: Recurrent dislocation of the patella treated by modified Roux-Goldthwait procedure. A prospective study of forty-seven knees. *J Bone Jt Surg* 1985;67-A:993–1005.

Additional Reading

Brown DE, Alexander AH, Lichtman DM: The Elmslie-Trillat procedure: Evaluation in patellar dislocation and subluxation. *Am J Sports Med* 1984;12:104–109.
Chrisman OD, Snook GS, Wilson TC: A long-term prospective study of the Hauser and Roux-Goldthwait procedures for recurrent patellar dislocation. *Clin Orthop* 1979;144:27–30.

Repair of Extensor Mechanism Injuries

14

Clarence L. Shields, Jr.

General Considerations

In most sports the extensor mechanism of the knee is repeatedly stressed. Some athletes will develop an inflammatory response from the accumulation of microtrauma, which can be concentrated at either the superior or inferior pole of the patella. This symptom complex has been well classified by Blazina and co-workers into several phases of jumper's knee.[1] Several studies have demonstrated the histological findings of tendon degeneration from the repeated microtrauma.[1-3] This process can remain localized to the attachments at either pole of the patella, as described by Phases 1 through 3 in Blazina's classification, or it can proceed to tendon failure in one catastrophic event.

Patellar Tendinitis Repair

Patients who have chronic tendinitis and do not respond to the treatment protocol outlined in our previous publication will require a surgical resection of the diseased portion of the tendon.[1]

Surgical Procedure and Techniques

As described by Bassett, the preferred approach to patellar tendinitis is to place the patient in a supine position and to apply a tourniquet to the upper thigh.[2] After localizing the tendon area, infiltrate the area over the inferior pole of the patella with 1 percent Xylocaine. Next, make a transverse incision in line with the skin creases for a distance of approximately 3 cm (Fig. 14-1b). Then, insert retractors to expose the patellar tendon. Again, note the exact area of tenderness by probing the patellar tendon with a forceps or hemostat.

Once the exact area of tenderness if noted, inject local anesthesia with 1 percent Xylocaine and split the patellar tendon longitudinally for a distance of about 2 cm. This maneuver usually reveals an area of grey granulation tissue and a disruption of the normal tendon architecture. Excise the abnormal area of patellar tendon in an elliptical fashion (Fig. 14-2). Now, curette the inferior pole of the patella and make, if necessary, several small drill holes into the tip of the patella to allow good bleeding to occur. Then, reapproximate

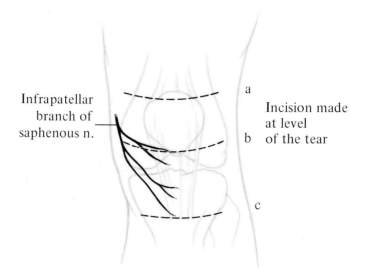

Infrapatellar
branch of
saphenous n.

Incision made
at level
of the tear

a

b

c

FIGURE 14-1. Incision is made at the level of lesion.

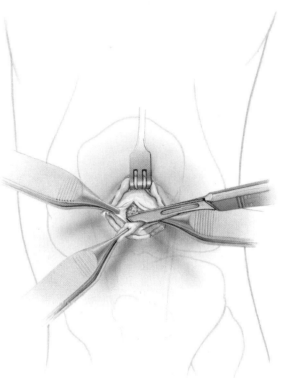

FIGURE 14-2

the defect in the patellar tendon by using #0 Vicryl suture. Finally, close
the skin and subcutaneous tissue in the usual fashion and apply a splint.

Postoperative Care and Rehabilitation

Protect the knee for a 3-week period. During this time, start isometric exercises
and then follow them by a full return to rehabilitation and function as indicated
below (Chap. 23).

Repair of Patellar Tendon Rupture

In the young athlete with open growth centers, an avulsion fracture of the tibial tuberosity happens when the quadriceps muscle fibers contract while the leg is forced into flexion. Typically, this rupture occurs when athletes land in the long-jump pit.

Complete failure of the extensor mechanism occurs in jumping sports such as basketball. Ruptures of the quadriceps mechanism happen in an older age group of athletes than do disruptions of the patellar tendon.[4,6] Also, in the case of older athletes, the prognosis for returning to normal function is not so good as it is in that of younger ones because of the high association of more extensive degenerative lesions in the tendon with chondromalacia of the patella.[5]

Surgical Procedure and Techniques

Place the patient in a supine position on the operating table, and raise the knee with a bolster to produce 30 degrees of flexion. Make a transverse incision over the level of the defect in the extensor mechanism (Fig. 14–1). Repair ruptures of either the superior or the inferior pole of the patella in the same manner by using #1 Ethibond suture. A complete disruption at the inferior pole is most common and the surgical technque for this injury will be described. Make a transverse incision over the level of the defect in the extensor mechanism (Fig. 14-1B).

After incising the skin dissect the subcutaneous tissue sharply with scissors to expose the infrapatellar branch of the saphenous nerve. Mobilize this sensory nerve for retraction during the procedure. Now, open the joint with the knife in the transverse plane at the inferior pole. This maneuver allows visualization of the articular surface of both medial and lateral facets of the patella. It is very important to document the amount and grade of chondromalacia present.

In order to reattach the tendon, it is necessary to orient properly the fibers to the pole of the patella. In doing so, it is useful to have your assistant lift the involved heel until the knee is in full extension. You can then approximate the normal attachment by grasping the tendon with a pair of forceps and pulling towards the patella. Mark both the center of the tendon and the inferior pole of the patella with methylene blue. Then, by replacing the heel on the bed, you will facilitate drilling in the proper direction because of the knee flexion.

Before drilling, place a saline-soaked sponge between the femoral groove and the patella to catch the bone fragments. Start with a $\frac{5}{64}$-inch drill bit close to the articular cartilage margin of the patella and in a direct line with the previously marked spot, while stabilizing the patella with the other hand. The drill will exit on the superior surface of the patella approximately 1.5 to 2 cm from the entry (Fig. 14-3). Drill parallel tunnels 1 cm apart from the central bone tunnel until the entire tendon can be repaired. Usually, 3 to 5 holes will encompass the whole tendon, and by ending with an odd number of tunnels, you will facilitate the suture tying over bony bridges.

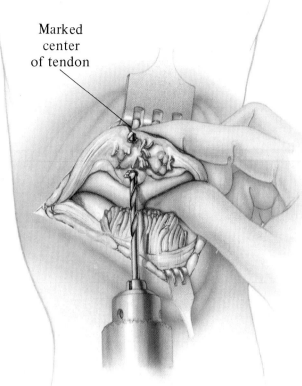

Marked
center
of tendon

FIGURE 14-3

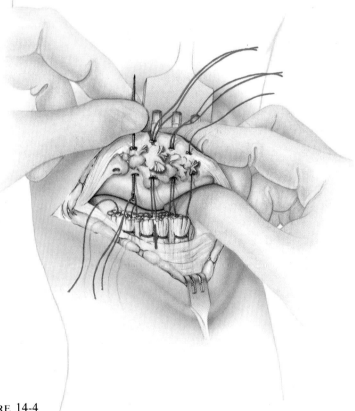

FIGURE 14-4

Place a #1 Ethibond suture in a horizontal mattress position beginning at the tendon edge. The first limb of the suture must be at the tendon center; then, turn medially before exiting at the free margin. Place a second suture adjacent to the first, but turn it laterally before exiting. Repeat this technique until the number of sutures is one less than the number of tunnels (Fig. 14-4).

108

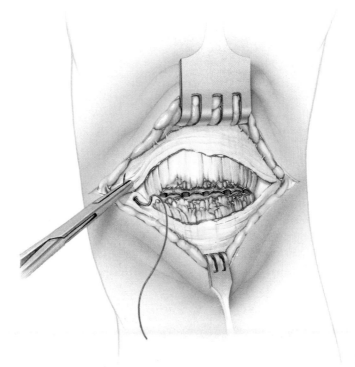

FIGURE 14-5

The central patellar hole will house the central limb of the first and second sutures. Pass these strands with a small straight Keith needle to exit on the superior surface of the patella. (The lateral and medial tunnels will have only one suture strand.) Now, place the knee bolster under the heel to produce recurvatum while the sutures are tied (Fig. 14-5). Be sure to range the knee from extension to 60 degrees of flexion before closure of the patellar retinaculum so that you can visualize the proper tracking of the extensor mechanism.

Repair tendon avulsions from the tibial tubercle by using a Richard's barbed staple. If there is a large bone fragment, then use an A-O cancellous screw with a soft tissue washer for fixation. It is very important to restore the proper tendon length; otherwise, patella may be too far proximally and a patellar tracking abnormality may develop.[5] Close the retinaculum with #0 Vicryl sutures on a tapered needle. The subcutaneous tissue is approximated with #3–0 Dexon and the skin is sutured with #4–0 clear nylon in a subcuticular fashion. Reinforce the final suturing with Steri-strips and place the patient in anterior-and-posterior-molded splints with the knee in full extension.

Postoperative Care and Rehabilitation

Allow the patient to ambulate and to bear weight as tolerated. Do not perform quadriceps exercises until 3 weeks have elapsed. At this point, place the patient in a hinged brace that will permit 0 to 45 degrees of knee flexion. This limited motion will aid in patellar cartilage nutrition. Maintain the immobilization for a total of 6 weeks; then, initiate our standard knee rehabilitation program with precautions against chondromalacia (Chap. 23).

References

1. Blazina ME, Kerlan RK, Jobe FW, et al: Jumper's knee. *Orthop Clin North Am* 1973;4:665–678.

2. Bassett F, Soucacos P, Carr W: Jumper's knee: Patellar tendinitis and patellar tendon rupture, in American Academy of Orthopedic Surgeons *Symposium on the Athlete's Knee.* St. Louis, Mosby, 1980.

3. Roels J, Martens M, Mulier JC, et al: Patellar tendinitis (Jumper's knee). *Am J Sports Med* 1978;6:362–368.

4. Siwek CW, Rao JP: Ruptures of the extensor mechanism of the knee joint. *J Bone Jt Surg* 1981;63-A:932–937.

5. Kelly DW, Carter VS, Jobe FW, et al: Patellar and quadriceps tendon ruptures—jumper's knee. *Am J Sports Med* 1984;12:375–380.

6. Martens M, Wouters P, Bursseens A, et al: Patellar tendinitis: Pathology and results of treatment. *Acta Orthop Scand* 1982;53:445–450.

Additional Reading

Feretti A, Ippolito E, et al: Jumper's knee. *Am J Sports Med* 1983;11:58–62.

Neckman JD, Alkire CC: Distal patellar pole fractures. A proposed common mechanism of injury. *Am J Sports Med* 1984;12:424–428.

Repair of Medial Collateral Ligament (MCL) Injuries

15

H. Royer Collins and Clarence L. Shields, Jr.

Acute MCL (Including Cruciate Ligament) Repair

General Considerations

Acute injuries to the medial side of the knee happen in all sports, but, in our practice, football proves to be the major contributor. These injuries usually occur when the athlete has a foot planted and then receives a valgus stress on the lateral side of his knee. There is also, in most cases, a component of external rotation applied at the knee. Usually, the patient feels a pop or tearing sensation on the medial side of the knee joint.

The deep and superficial portions of the medial collateral ligaments may be torn above the joint line, at the joint line, or below it. Both layers may be disrupted at the same level or at different levels. The anterior cruciate may also be torn along with the lateral capsule and menisci. Occasionally, the force may be so severe as to include the posterior cruciate ligament, which can result in a complete knee dislocation.

Examine the injured knee gently with abduction and adduction stress tests along with a Lachman and a posterior drawer test. Compare the test results with those of the normal extremity to determine the amount of instability. Before any stress testing, be sure to relax the patient's hamstrings. To do so, a local anesthetic and gentle massage of the muscles may be necessary. On occasion, this may necessitate an examination of the knee under general anesthesia.

Valgus instability with full extension indicates a more severe injury that includes the posterior capsule. Valgus laxity with 30 degrees of knee flexion indicates a medial collateral ligament Grade III sprain whenever no definite endpoint can be felt.

Gentle palpation along the ligament for maximum tenderness is helpful in locating the level of the tear. Also, immediately after the injury, a defect in the ligament can be seen while stress testing. The study of Indelicato shows that Grade III sprains with intact cruciate ligaments and normal menisci can be treated with a hinged cast or brace.[1] It is our policy to arthroscope all complete tears and to repair surgically those that involve the medial meniscus at the joint line.[2]

A positive Lachman test and a pivot shift indicate damage to the anterior cruciate ligament and possibly to the lateral capsule. Evaluate the posterior

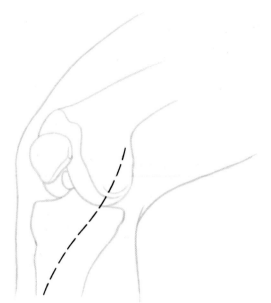

FIGURE 15-1

cruciate with a posterior drawer test; also, be sure to look for a posterior drop back or a sag sign.

Surgical Procedure and Techniques

Repeat stress testing of both knees after the patient is anesthetized. After routine prep and drape, begin the skin incision at the level of the medial femoral epicondyle (Fig. 15-1), and run it obliquely towards the attachment of the pes anserinus tendons on the tibia. Next, undermine the subcutaneous tissue anteriorly to the medial patellar border. Posteriorly, develop the skinflap until the saphenous nerve is located. In doing so, take care to avoid injury to the infrapatellar branch of the saphenous nerve.

The areas of the hemorrhage correspond to the injury levels along the medial collateral ligament. Identify the lower edge of the vastus medialis muscle fibers at the patella, and palpate the medial border of the articular cartilage of the medial femoral condyle along the intercondylar notch. In making the anterior capsular incision, follow this articular cartilage margin to the level of the meniscus. This path will avoid injury to the fat pad.

Open the synovium along the same line and irrigate the joint with Garamycin solution. To probe both the anterior cruciate ligament (ACL) and posterior cruciate ligament (PCL), use a Dandy nerve hook and note any hemorrhage within the fibers (Fig. 15-2). If you now apply valgus stress to the joint, the medial compartment will open, and you can visualize well the posterior horn of the medial meniscus.

Start the posterior capsular incision at the soft spot in the capsule, just behind the medial femoral condyle, and continue it to the top of the pes anserinus tendons. In making this cut, follow the course of the posterior edge of the superficial medial collateral ligament. Also, by reflecting the retinaculum between the anterior and posterior capsular incisions, you will allow for adequate suture placement between the two capsular incisions. Keep this cut parallel to the lower border of vastus medialis muscle and involve only the superficial retinaculum. Use scissors to free this layer from the deep portion of the medial collateral ligament for a distance of 1 cm below the joint line (Fig. 15-3).

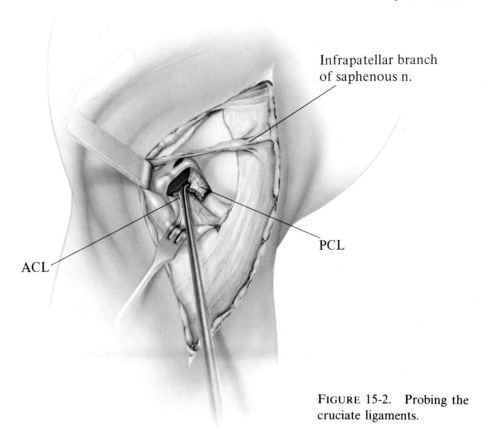

Infrapatellar branch
of saphenous n.

PCL

ACL

FIGURE 15-2. Probing the
cruciate ligaments.

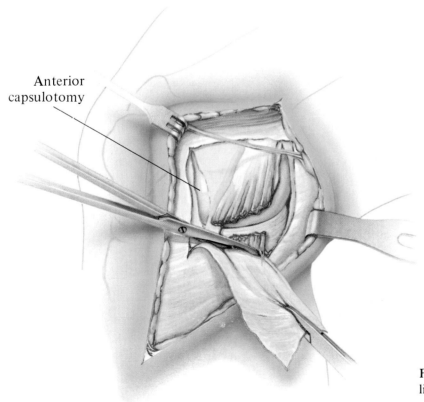

Anterior
capsulotomy

FIGURE 15-3. Medial collateral
ligament torn at the joint line.

113

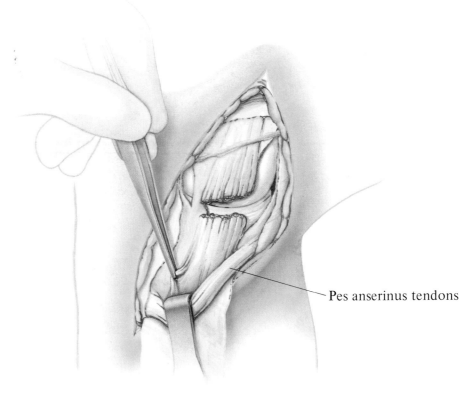

Pes anserinus tendons

FIGURE 15-4

At this point, stop and look for the extent of the tear. Now retract the pes anserinus tendon distally with a United States Army (USA) retractor to allow visualization of the attachment of the superficial fibers to the periosteum of the tibia. Grasp the ligament with forceps and pull it towards the joint line to verify its continuity (Fig. 15-4). In the proximal limb, probe the meniscotibial and meniscofemoral portions anterior and posterior to the capsular opening. Now, start the repair at the posterior apex of the tear, provided the cruciate ligaments are intact (Fig. 15-9). If one or both are torn, delay collateral ligament repair until you have placed the cruciate ligament sutures. This allows you to take advantage of the increased exposure provided by the valgus instability.

You can extend the anterior capsular incision proximally to allow more exposure in the notch. To repair midsubstance tears in the anterior cruciate ligament, use horizontal mattress sutures and #0 cottony Dacron on a small cutting needle. In doing so, attempt to orient the anteromedial and posterolateral bundles of the ligament. To repair tears from the femoral insertion, use a Bunnell stitch with the cottony Dacron in each bundle. It is imperative that sutures exit at the end of the ligament stump. Finally, curette the avulsion site down to bleeding bone.

The augmentation of anterior cruciate ligament repairs with patellar tendon increases the chances of successful repair, as Cabaud and Feagin have shown.[3] The purpose of this graft is primarily for vascularity and only a small increase in repair strength can be expected. The size of this graft is thus smaller than the graft utilized for reconstruction of the anterior cruciate ligament.

Detach a strip of patellar tendon 5 mm wide from the medial border of the patella, but leave it attached to the tibia. Push a large curved clamp beneath the fat pad to exit just anterior to the transverse meniscal ligament.

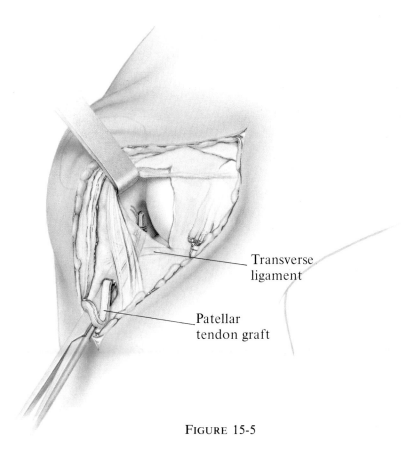

Transverse ligament

Patellar tendon graft

FIGURE 15-5

Using #0 cottony Dacron, place two sutures in a Bunnell fashion to exit at the free end of the graft and pass the graft under the fat pad (Fig. 15-5). Now, flex the knee into the figure-of-four position and drill a $\frac{3}{32}$-inch smooth Steinmann pin from the notch towards the lateral femoral epicondyle until it tents the skin laterally. Then, rotate the hip internally while holding the knee flexion constant in order to avoid bending the pin. Next, develop the Ellison iliotibial band transfer (Chap. 18). If the pin is at the upper border of the iliotibial band, then proximal retraction of the transfer will allow the exit site of the pin to be visible. If the pin tract is too anterior, a separate incision can be made in the fascia of the vastus lateralis muscle. In this latter case, curette the periosteum in order to visualize the exit hole. Finally, remove the pin with the drill and make a second and parallel hole 3 to 5 cm from the first (Fig. 15-6).

If the posterior cruciate is torn, place two Bunnell stitches of cottony Dacron in the ligament. A tibial avulsion can be repaired by drilling two parallel holes in an anteroposterior direction.[4,5] An interval is developed at the posteromedial corner between the capsule and the medial head of the gastrocnemius. This interval allows a malleable retractor to be placed anterior to the muscle for protection of the neurovascular bundle. Place the index finger at the origin site posteriorly and start drilling with a smooth $\frac{3}{32}$ Steinmann pin 1 cm medial to the patellar tendon so that it exits on the posterior tibial surface approximately 1 cm below the joint surface. Drill a second hole that is 3 to 5 mm medially away from the first. In doing so, be careful not to damage the patellar tendon augmentation graft (Fig. 15-7). If necessary, the posterior capsule may be cut vertically where the cruciate enters the joint. This maneuver will permit curetting of the origin site and also allow better retrieval of the suture passer, which is inserted anteriorly.

115

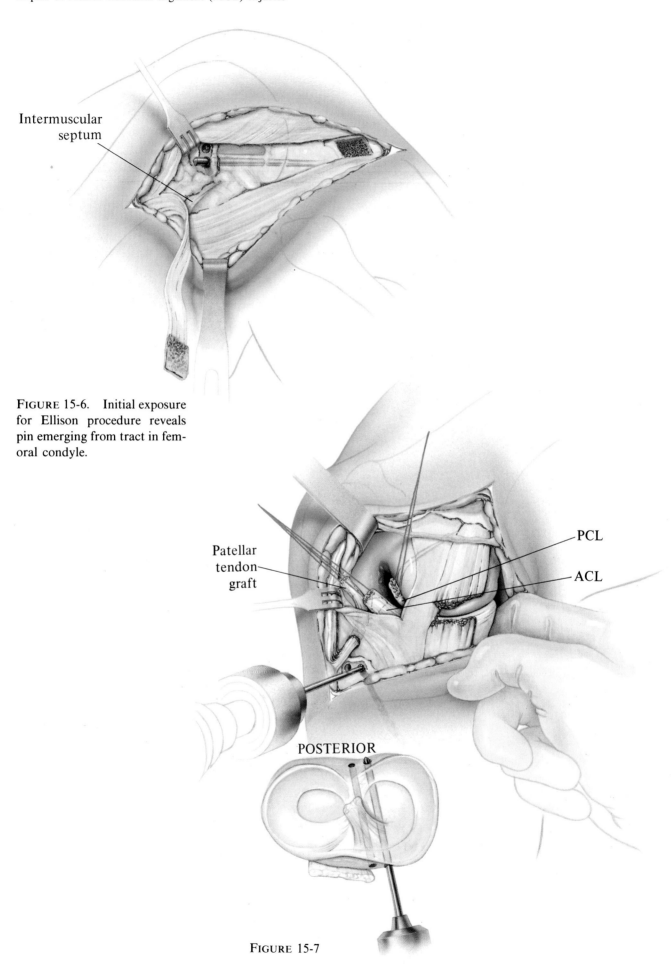

Intermuscular septum

FIGURE 15-6. Initial exposure for Ellison procedure reveals pin emerging from tract in femoral condyle.

Patellar tendon graft

PCL

ACL

POSTERIOR

FIGURE 15-7

116

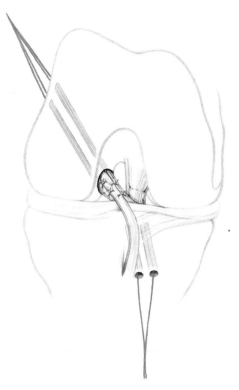

FIGURE 15-8. Positions of anterior cruciate ligament and posterior cruciate ligament repairs in the notch with patellar tendon augmentation sutured to the anterior cruciate ligament.

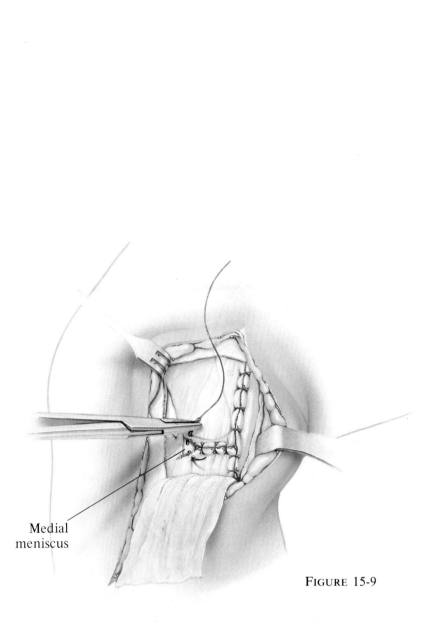

Medial meniscus

FIGURE 15-9

Pass a strand from each suture through the drill holes. Now, apply tension anteriorly and check the posterior cruciate ligament for fiber orientation and proper position. Next, separate the sutures in the anterior cruciate ligament from the strands in the patellar tendon graft. Thread the Richards' suture passer from the lateral femoral condyle and pass the two strands of the cruciate ligament and the one from the graft through each drill hole. Be sure to check the tension and fiber orientation in the anterior cruciate ligament (Fig. 15-8).

Start the repair of the posterior capsule tear and the medial collateral at the posterior apex. Using a tapered needle, place #0 Vicryl sutures in the femoral side of the ligament, the periphery of the meniscus, and the tibial attachment. Take care not to advance the ligament anteriorly because, if you do so, the medial meniscus will then fold in on itself. Tie these sutures after placement (Fig. 15-9). Next, repair the superficial portion of the ligament to the periosteum of the tibia by pulling distally to restore its length and then

117

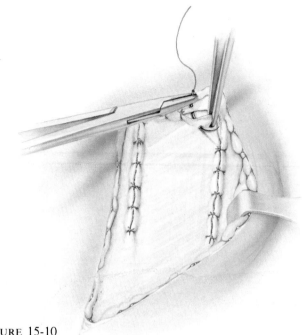

FIGURE 15-10

by suturing rather than stapling it. A staple near the pes tendons will produce inflammation and require removal at a later date. Also, avoid placing sutures in the anterior free margin of the superficial collateral ligament because these will inhibit its normal excursion with knee flexion. Repair the retinaculum with the same suture (Fig. 15-10).

Now, tie the posterior cruciate sutures while pulling the tibia anteriorly. Next, tie the anterior cruciate sutures. The graft will now lay directly on top of the ligament, as indicated in Figure 15-8. Use #4–0 Vicryl to anchor the graft's position on the ligament. Irrigate the joint with Garamycin solution and close the synovium with #3–0 Dexon. Repair the capsule and retinaculum with #0 Vicryl and the subcutaneous tissue with #3–0 Dexon and the skin with #4–0 nylon by using a subcuticular technique.

Postoperative Care and Rehabilitation

Immobilize the knee with 30 degrees of flexion in a cylinder cast with neutral rotation of the tibia. After 2 weeks, change the patient to a hinged cast with the range of motion limited from 40 to 80 degrees. Have the patient continue a nonweightbearing ambulation for 1 month postsurgery. At 4 weeks, remove the flexion stop and allow the patient to bear weight as tolerated. After 6 weeks have elapsed, remove the cast and, if only the anterior cruciate ligament is involved, outfit the patient with a temporary brace. Have him wear a 40-degree extension stop and allow him full flexion if only the anterior cruciate was repaired. When both anterior and posterior cruciate ligaments were repaired, block flexion at 120 degrees. The rehabilitation is started as outlined in Chapter 23 for the anterior and/or posterior cruciate ligaments.

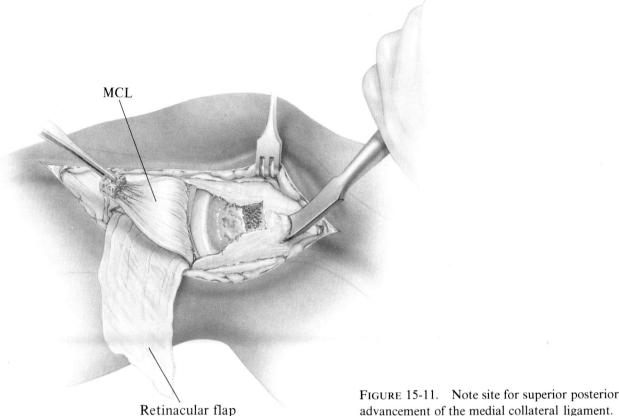

MCL

Retinacular flap

FIGURE 15-11. Note site for superior posterior advancement of the medial collateral ligament.

Chronic MCL Repair

General Considerations

In the patient with chronic medial collateral ligament (MCL) instability of the knee, several procedures are available, depending on where the site of the original injury is located.[6-8] If the laxity occurs proximal to the meniscus, there has been a stretching or tearing of the tissues between the femoral attachment and the joint line, and advancement of the medial collateral ligament is carried proximally. Occasionally, the valgus instability is associated with anterior and rotational instability, and an anterior cruciate ligament reconstruction may be combined with the medial reconstruction.

Surgical Procedure and Techniques

After routine prep and drape, use a utility medial incision that starts at the medial femoral epicondyle and extends down towards the tibial crest (Fig. 15-1). Retract the retinaculum to expose distally the medial capsular structures and the superficial medial collateral ligament. (Frequently, this is all combined in one mass of scar tissue.) Base the reconstruction on the Nicholas 5–1 procedure, which osteotomizes the proximal attachment of the medial collateral ligament from the adductor tubercle.[9]

Start the incision for the Nicholas procedure in the posteromedial capsule at the posterior margin of the posterior oblique ligament. Make another anterior incision over the anterior edge of the medial collateral ligament. Then, retract this detached strip of superficial collateral ligament and the deep collateral ligament distally to the joint line (Fig. 15-11). Inspect the meniscus and

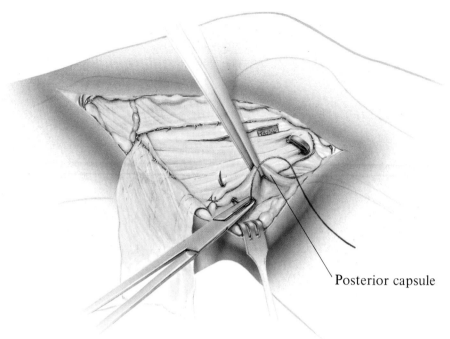

Posterior capsule

FIGURE 15-12

the interior of the joint, and if the patient is found to have damage to the meniscus, remove the meniscal tear at this time. If, however, the anterior cruciate ligament is not functioning, then carry out a reconstruction of the ligament at this time (see Chap. 18, Repair of Chronic Anterior Cruciate Ligament [ACL] Injuries).

Be sure to advance the attachment of the medial collateral ligament proximally and slightly posterior to its original attachment and hold it in its new bed with a barbed Richards' staple. With the knee in 45 degrees of flexion, imbricate the posterior capsule over the posterior oblique portion of the medial collateral ligament with #0 Vicryl. This will tighten the laxity of the posterior medial side of the joint (Fig. 15-12). Now, dissect the semimembranosus tendon proximally along the muscle belly until the tendon can be advanced over the new insertion site of the medial collateral ligament (Fig. 15-13). Next, suture the tendon to the ligament with #0 Vicryl sutures to further reinforce the posterior medial corner of the joint.

At this point in the operation, test the knee to see if stability has been achieved. If not, then diessect the sartorius (tailor's) muscle free, transfer it anteriorly, and attach it to the medial collateral ligament as described by Slocum, Larson, and James.[6] This again reinforces the medial collateral ligament.

Insert a Reliavac drain and close the capsule with interrupted #0 Vicryl. Suture the subcutaneous tissue with #3–0 Dexon and the skin with #4–0 subcuticular nylon.

Postoperative Care and Rehabilitation

Immobilize the knee with molded splints, anteriorly and posteriorly, in a position of 45 degrees of flexion. Start full weightbearing ambulation on the day following surgery as well as isometric quadriceps and hamstring setting exercises. At 2 weeks, remove the splints and apply a hinged cast with a 20-degree extension stop and allow the patient full flexion. Continue the immo-

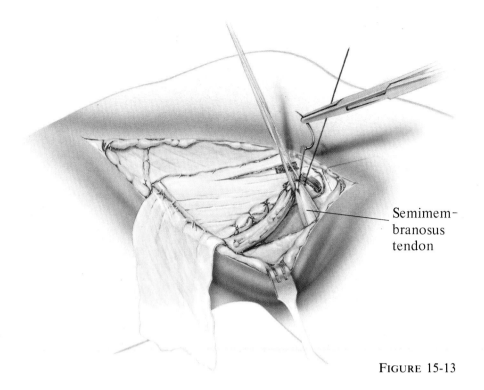

Semimem-
branosus
tendon

FIGURE 15-13

bilization for a total of 6 weeks, at which time remove the cast and start the patient's rehabilitation in a temporary brace. Start the rehabilitation according to the medial collateral ligament protocol (Chap. 23).

References

Acute MCL (Including Cruciate Ligament) Repair

1. Indelicato PA: Non-operative treatment of complete tears of the medial collateral ligament. *J Bone Jt Surg* 1983;65-A:323–329.
2. Price CT, Allen WC: Ligament repair in the knee with preservation of the meniscus. *J Bone Jt Surg* 1978;60-A:61–65.
3. Cabaud HE, Feagin JA, et al: Acute anterior cruciate ligament injury and augmented repair. Experimental studies. *Am J Sports Med* 1980;8:395–401.
4. Bianchi M: Acute tears of the posterior cruciate ligament: Clinical study and results of operative treatment in 27 cases. *Am J Sports Med* 1983;11:308–314.
5. Larson RL: Combined instabilities of the knee. *Clin Orthop* 1980;147:68–75.

Chronic MCL Repair

6. Slocum DB, Larson RL, James SL: Late reconstruction of ligamentous injuries of the medial compartment of the knee. *Clin Orthop* 1974;100:23–55.
7. Larson RL: Dislocations and ligamentous injuries of the knee, in Rockwood CA, Green DP (eds): *Fractures.* Philadelphia, Lippincott, 1975, zv, pp xxil, 92, 1495.
8. Slocum DB, Larson RL: Pes anserinus transplantation; a surgical procedure for control of rotatory instability of the knee. *J Bone Jt Surg* 1968;50-A:226–242.
9. Nicholas JA: The five-one reconstruction for anteromedial instability of the knee; indications, technique, and the results in fifty-two patients. *J Bone Jt Surg* 1973;55-A:899–922.

Additional Reading

Feagin JA: Operative treatment of acute and chronic knee problems. *Clin Sports Med* 1985;4:325–321.

121

Hughston JC, Barrett GR: Acute anteromedial rotatory instability. Long-term results of surgical repair. *J Bone Jt Surg* 1983;65-A:145–153.

Indelicato PA, Bittar ES: A perspective of lesions associated with ACL insufficiency of the knee, a review of 100 cases. *Clin Orthop* 1985;198:77–80.

Kennedy JC: Application of prosthetics to anterior cruciate ligament reconstruction and repair. *Clin Orthop* 1983;172:125–128.

Noyes FR: Intra-articular cruciate reconstruction. I: Perspectives on graft strength, vascularization, and immediate motion after replacement. *Clin Orthop* 1983;172:71–77.

Noyes FR, McGinness GH: Controversy about treatment of the knee anterior cruciate laxity. *Clin Orthop* 1985;198:61–76.

Simonet WT, Sim FH: Current concepts in the treatment of ligamentous instability of the knee. *Mayo Clin Proc* 1984;59:67–76.

Snook GA: A short history of the anterior cruciate ligament and treatment of tears. *Clin Orthop* 1983;172:11–13.

Repair of Lateral Collateral Ligament (LCL) Injuries

16

H. Royer Collins and Clarence L. Shields, Jr.

Acute LCL Repair

General Considerations

Although they are far less frequent than injuries to the medial side of the joint, injuries to the lateral supporting structures may also occur in athletes. These injuries are a result of varus and rotational forces against the medial side of the joint.

There are several diagnostic findings. If the posterior capsule is involved, there may be observable varus laxity with the knee in full extension. If the anterolateral capsule is involved, there may evidence of a lateral pivot shift indicating anterolateral rotatory instability. If the posterolateral capsule (including the arcuate complex) is involved, the external rotation recurvatum test as described by Hughston is positive.[1,2] There will also be some posterolateral subluxation detectable when the knee is flexed and the tibia is rotated laterally and pushed posteriorly. In this type of injury, also look for damage to the peroneal nerve and assess the peroneal function for impairment.

Surgical Procedure and Techniques

For a distance of approximately 15 cm, make a lateral utility incision starting at the lateral femoral epicondyle and in line with the iliotibial band, extending just distal to Gerdy's tubercle (Fig. 16-1). Next, expose the iliotibial band

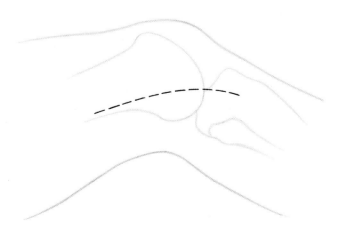

FIGURE 16-1

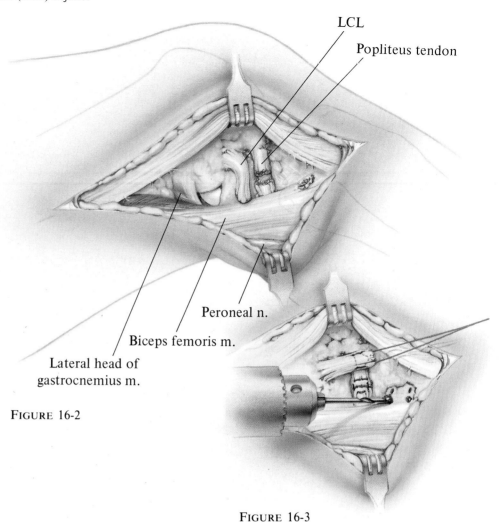

LCL

Popliteus tendon

Peroneal n.

Biceps femoris m.

Lateral head of
gastrocnemius m.

FIGURE 16-2

FIGURE 16-3

and carry the dissection posteriorly to expose the head of the fibula, the attachment of the biceps femoris, and the entire posterolateral joint. Take care not to injure the peroneal nerve, particularly proximally in the wound where it is in intimate contact with the biceps femoris and the entire posterior lateral joint. The popliteus tendon as well as the entire arcuate complex and the lateral head of the gastrocnemius can be easily visualized (Fig. 16-2).

If there is any question about the lateral meniscus, make a lateral incision into the joint so this can be well visualized. If necessary in order to get exposure, detach the iliotibial band from Gerdy's tubercle with a fragment of bone so that it can be reattached with a staple. This will allow exploration of the anterior and posterior cruciate ligaments. The cruciate repair is outlined in Chap. 15.)

The anterior capsule may be repaired with #0 Vicryl on a cutting needle if it is torn. Then, suture back all tendinous and ligamentous structures with #1 Ethibond suture. If the fibular collateral ligament, the popliteus muscle, or the lateral head of the gastrocnemius and capsule are torn from their insertion into the femur, reattach them with a staple. If the lateral collateral ligament is torn from its distal attachment into the head of the fibula, place drill holes into the fibula and then reattach the ligament (Fig. 16-3). With the knee flexed, the posterior capsule is repaired with interrupted #0 Vicryl (Fig. 16-4). During the repair of all these structures, it is important to avoid excessive retraction of the peroneal nerve.

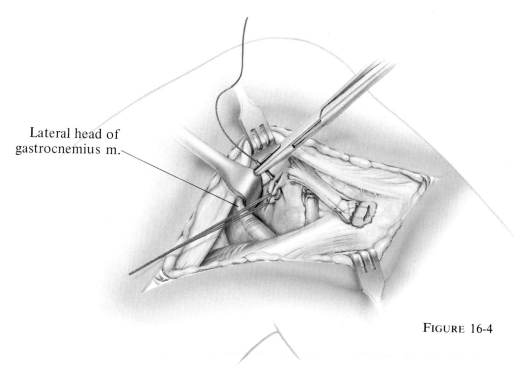

Lateral head of
gastrocnemius m.

FIGURE 16-4

If there is evidence of peroneal nerve dysfunction on the initial physical examination, isolate the peroneal nerve through this exposure by dissecting farther subcutaneously and by extending the skin incision farther distally. Then, follow the nerve from its position in contact with the biceps femoris to its course around the neck of the fibula and determine the extent of damage. If the nerve is in continuity, no further surgery need be done. If, however, the nerve is completely severed, repair it by using microsurgical techniques. Following closure of all of these structures, including the subcutaneous tissue and the skin, apply anterior and posterior plaster splints with 45 degrees of knee flexion.

Postoperative Care and Rehabilitation

The patient is kept nonweightbearing for 14 days. Start isometric quadriceps and hamstring setting exercises as soon as the patient tolerates them. At 2 weeks, place the patient in a hinged cast with the knee range limited at 30 to 90 degrees. If the peroneal nerve was injured, add a foot plate to the cast to control the foot drop. Remove the cast at 6 weeks and initiate the knee rehabilitation program. (Chap. 23).

Chronic LCL Repair

General Considerations

In the patient presenting with chronic lateral collateral ligament instability, one has to determine whether there is anterolateral instability, posterolateral instability, or a combination of them. In the patient with anterolateral instability, several procedures may be used. Since this is frequently associated with anterior cruciate ligament insufficiency in severe cases, extra-articular repairs are combined with intra-articular reconstruction. However, in the less severe

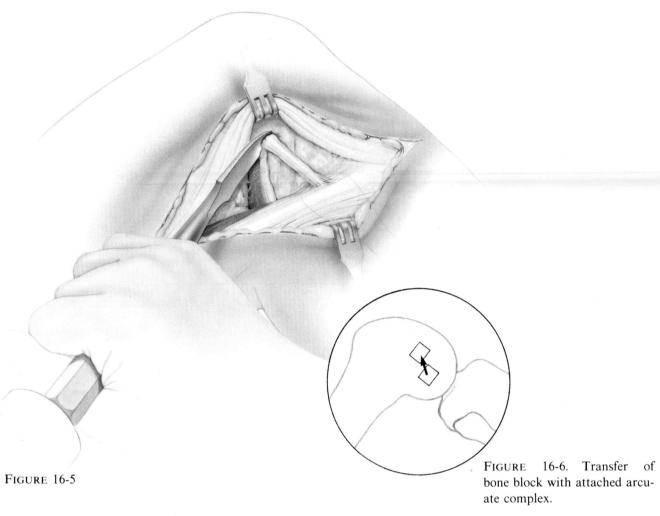

FIGURE 16-5

FIGURE 16-6. Transfer of bone block with attached arcuate complex.

case, extra-articular repair alone may be all that is needed. This is described in Chapter 18.

Surgical Procedure and Techniques

If the patient presents with chronic posterolateral instability as evidenced by a positive external rotation recurvatum test and by posterolateral laxity, then carry out reconstruction of the posterolateral corner of the joint as described by Baker, Norwood and Hughston.[3] Use the lateral utility incision to expose the posterolateral corner of the joint (Fig. 16-1). Osteotomize the lateral collateral ligament, popliteus tendon, lateral head of the gastrocnemius, and the adherent posterolateral capsule from the lateral femoral condyle (Fig. 16-5). Then, create a new site superiorly and slightly anteriorly, advance the structures as one unit, and staple them into the new bed with the knee held in 90 degrees of flexion (Fig. 16-6). Be sure to correct all intra-articular pathology prior to the repositioning of this complex.

As mentioned previously, if it is necessary to detach a portion of the iliotibial band with a fragment of bone from Gerdy's tubercle in order to get exposure, do this and then reattach the iliotibial band after repair is accomplished. (Follow the technique described in Chap. 18 on the Ellison procedure.) Now, expose the attachment of the biceps femoris into the fibular head, and detach from the fibular head the portion of the biceps femoris attachment that is lateral to the lateral collateral ligament. Release this portion proximally to allow advancement of the biceps femoris, which is then advanced to near

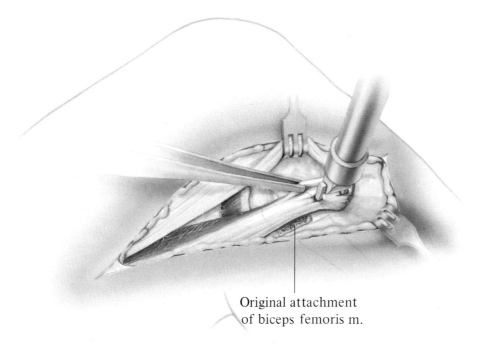

Original attachment of biceps femoris m.

FIGURE 16-7. Tibia is rotated externally.

Gerdy's tubercle. Next, with the knee in 90 degrees of flexion and external rotation, staple the biceps femoris tendon to its new attachment (Fig. 16-7). This detachment and reattachment gives further dynamic reinforcement to the posterolateral repair of the joint.

Before closing, if the capsule is found to be loose, tighten it prior to passing the strip of iliotibial band under the lateral collateral ligament and tightening it. Close the subcutaneous tissue with absorbable sutures and the skin with #4–0 clear nylon.

Postoperative Care and Rehabilitation

After closure of the wound, place the knee in 60 degrees of flexion with external rotation of the tibia and apply a cast. Start rehabilitation with the isometric exercises that avoid stressing the biceps femoris and those tendons that have been transferred. At 6 weeks, remove the cast and institute routine knee rehabilitation (Chap. 23).

References

1. Hughston JC, Norwood LA: The posterolateral drawer test and external rotational recurvatum test for posterolateral rotatory instability of the knee. *Clin Orthop* 1980;147:82–87.
2. Baker CL, Norwood LA, Hughston JC: Acute posterolateral rotatory instability of the knee. *J Bone Jt Surg* 1983;65-A:614–618.
3. Baker CL, Norwood LA, Hughston JC: Acute combined posterior cruciate and posterolateral instability of the knee. *Am J Sports Med* 1984;12:204–208.

Additional Reading

DeLee JC, Riley MB, Rockwood CA: Acute straight lateral instability of the knee. *Am J Sports* 1983;11:404–411.
Losee RE, Johnson TR, Southwick WO: Anterior subluxation of the lateral tibial plateau, a diagnostic test and operative repair. *J Bone Jt Surg* 1978;60-A:1015–1030.
MacIntosh DL, Darby TA: Lateral substitution reconstruction. *J Bone Jt Surg* 1976;58-B:142.

17 Repair of Posterior Cruciate Ligament (PCL) Injuries

H. Royer Collins and Clarence L. Shields, Jr.

Acute PCL Repair

General Considerations

The posterior cruciate ligament is the primary restraint to the posterior displacement of the tibia, and along with the posterior capsule, it also resists internal rotation of the tibia. Studies have shown that as the tibia rotates internally in terminal extension, tension in the posterior cruciate ligament increases. Injuries to the posterior cruciate ligament complex may occur either as a result of force against the anterior tibia when the knee is in the flexed position or as a result of hyperextension. This injury can also be associated with severe medial or lateral collateral ligament injuries.

Clinical evaluation does not always reveal positive posterior drawer sign; hence diagnosis may be difficult. If damage to the posterior cruciate ligament occurs in association with collateral ligament injury, the patient will frequently demonstrate varus or valgus instability when the knee is out in full extension.[2,3] A posterior sag sign may be present when the knees and hips are flexed to 90 degrees and the examiner looks from the side. In these instances, X-rays may be helpful if the cruciate ligament has been avulsed with a piece of bone from the tibia.

Surgical Procedure and Techniques

Limited arthroscopy may be beneficial to identify the tear in the posterior cruciate ligament; however, one must be careful to avoid excessive amount of fluid installation. Since the posterior capsule is ruptured, there is a strong possibility of fluid extravasation into the popliteal fossa.

The surgical approach to the posterior cruciate ligament is through the anteromedial utility incision (Fig. 17-1). This incision, which we described in discussing medial repairs (Chap. 15), allows the entire posteromedial and posterior side of the joint to be visualized. Next, make a medial parapatellar capsular incision to determine the status of the posterior cruciate ligament along with the menisci and the anterior cruciate ligament. (Repair midsubstance tears as described in the repair of the anterior cruciate ligament injuries; see Chap. 15.)

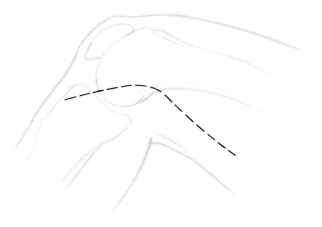

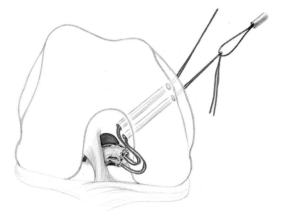

FIGURE 17-1   FIGURE 17-2

If the posterior cruciate ligament is torn from its tibial insertion, incise the posterior capsule longitudinally behind the posterior oblique ligament to obtain further exposure. In order to get more exposure in the posterior medial corner of the joint, release a portion of the attachment of the medial head of the gastrocnemius. This maneuver will expose the posterior horn of the medial meniscus as well as the attachment of the posterior cruciate ligament.

Place the sutures in the posterior cruciate ligament as described in the repair associated with medial collateral ligament injuries (Chap. 15). If the posterior cruciate ligament has been avulsed from the medial femoral condyle, make two drill holes through the medial femoral condyle and exit into the joint at the area of insertion of the posterior cruciate ligament (Fig. 17-2). Now, place four sutures of #0 cottony Dacron in the posterior cruciate ligament in a Bunnell technique by bringing the sutures out through the two drill holes. Be sure to allow for correct orientation of the fiber bundles of the posterior cruciate ligament. Finally, tie the sutures over the medial femoral epicondyle.

Repair the posterior capsule and the medial head of the gastrocnemius with interrupted #0 Vicryl sutures. Close the synovium anteriorly with running #3-0 Dexon and the capsule with interrupted #0 Vicryl. Use #3-0 Dexon for the subcutaneous tissue. Close the skin with a subcuticular #4-0 clear nylon and reinforce with Steri-strips. Immobilize the knee in full extension with molded splints, anteriorly and posteriorly.

Chronic PCL Repair

General Considerations

The patient with chronic instability of the cruciate ligament has difficulty with "giving away," climbing hills, and particularly in going down hills. The patient usually exhibits a significant posterior drawer and occasionally may have a positive external rotation recurvatum test for posterior lateral instability of the knee.[4] In the patient with combined instabilities, the medial head of the gastrocnemius transfer is combined with an arcuate complex advancement as described in chronic lateral ligament instability (Chap. 16).[5,6]

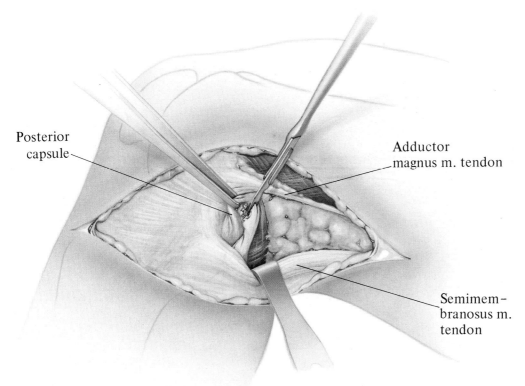

Posterior capsule

Adductor magnus m. tendon

Semimem-branosus m. tendon

FIGURE 17-3

Surgical Procedure and Techniques

Use a medial utility incision to expose the medial head of the gastrocnemius (Fig. 17-1). Release the tendinous portion of the medial head of the gastrocnemius from the femur, but leave the muscular attachment intact. It is important to start the release as close to the femur as possible in order to gain sufficient length of the tendon for transfer (Fig. 17-3). Next, strip the tendinous portion distally for a distance of 5 to 6 cm below the joint line (Fig. 17-4). Identify the posterior capsule while the gastrocnemius is being retracted posteriorly to protect the neurovascular structures.

After a sufficient length of tendon has been obtained, make a median parapatellar incision in the capsule. Then, pass a curved clamp anteriorly to penetrate the posterior capsule in the area where the posterior cruciate ligament normally enters (Fig. 17-5). Enlarge the posterior capsular hole with a #15 blade knife, being careful to protect the neurovascular structures. Into the tendinous portion of the medial head of the gastrocnemius, place a Bunnell stitch of umbilical tape by inserting a Gallie needle and then by pulling it through the posterior capsule into the joint.

Now, place the knee in 90 degrees of flexion and dorsiflex the ankle. At this point, determine whether the tendon is long enough to insert into the femur. If not, suture a leader of Dacron tape into the tendon in a Bunnell fashion. Next, start a smooth Steinmann pin just above the insertion of the medial collateral ligament on the medial femoral condyle. Aim it to exit at the origin of the posterior cruciate ligament in the anterior condylar notch. After the position is accurate, enlarge the hole to ⅜ths of an inch (Fig. 17-6).

Finally, pull umbilical tape in the tendinous portion of the medial head of the gastrocnemius through the posterior capsule. It is very important to make sure that the tendinous portion does come through the posterior capsule and is exposed in the joint. Push the suture passer through the drill hole

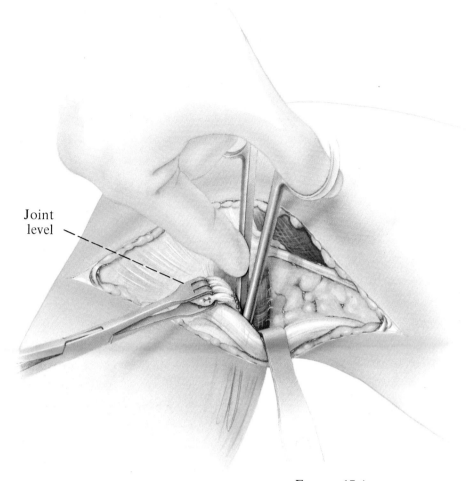

Joint level

FIGURE 17-4

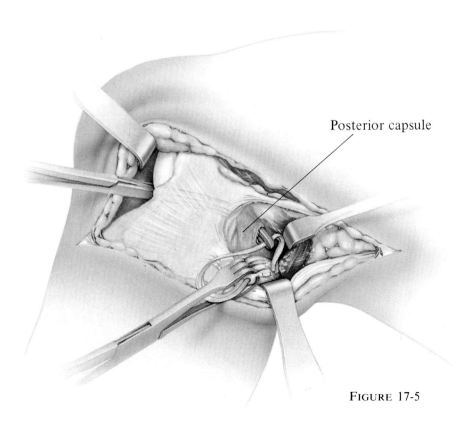

Posterior capsule

FIGURE 17-5

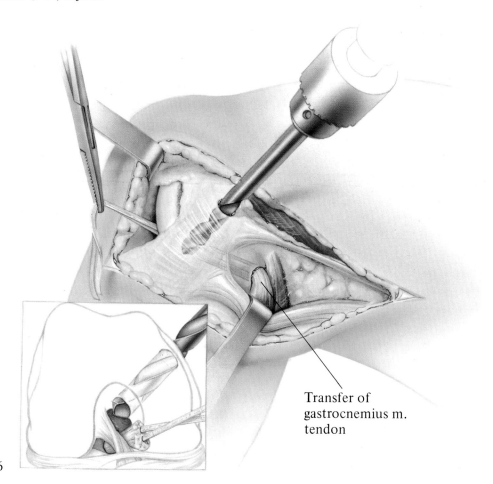

Transfer of
gastrocnemius m.
tendon

FIGURE 17-6

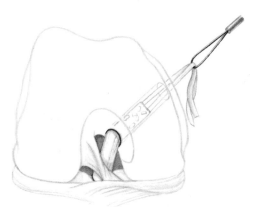

FIGURE 17-7

from the medial side into the notch. Be sure to pull the tendon into the femoral tunnel while keeping the knee in flexion and reducing the tibia anteriorly. This maneuver assures that there is a sufficient amount of tendon within the bone tunnel (Fig. 17-7). Staple the tape near the opening at the femoral condyle.

Irrigate the joint with Garamycin solution and close the anterior medial capsular incision: the synovium with #3–0 Dexon and the capsule with interrupted #0 Vicryl. Leave the posterior capsular incision open. Close subcutaneous tissue with #3–0 Dexon and the skin with #4–0 subcuticular nylon reinforced with Steri-strips.

Postoperative Care and Rehabilitation

Place the knee in molded splints, anteriorly and posteriorly, and in 40 degrees of flexion. Start ambulation, nonweightbearing, and maintain during the first 2 weeks. After this period of time, place the patient in a cylinder cast at 45 degrees of knee flexion and allow weightbearing as tolerated. At 6 weeks, remove the limb from its immobilization and start the patient on a rehabilitation program designed to emphasize quadriceps and calf-muscle exercises (Chap. 23).

References

1. Girgis FG, Marshall JL, et al: The cruciate ligaments of the knee joint. Anatomical, functional and experimental analysis. *Clin Orthop* 1975;106:216–231.
2. Hughston JC, Bowden JA, et al: Acute tears of the posterior cruciate ligament. Results of operative treatment. *J Bone Jt Surg* 1980;62G2-A:438–450.
3. Hughston JC, Degenhardt TC: Reconstruction of the posterior cruciate ligament. *Clin Orthop* 1982:164:59–77.
4. Hughston JC, Norwood LA: The posterolateral drawer test and external rotational recurvatum test for posterolateral instability of the knee. *Clin Orthop* 1980;147:82–87.
5. Insall JN, Hood RW: Bone block transfer of the medial head of the gastrocnemius for posterior cruciate insufficiency. *J Bone Jt Surg* 1982;64-A:691–699.
6. Kennedy JC, Galpin RD: The use of the medial head of the gastrocnemius muscle in the posterior cruciate deficient knee. Indications—technique—results. *Am J Sports Med* 1982;10:63–74.

Additional Reading

Acute PCL Repair

Bianchi M: Acute tears of the posterior cruciate ligament. Clinical study and results of operative treatment in 27 cases. *Am J Sports Med* 1983;11:308–314.
DeLee JC, Riley MB, Rockwood CA: Acute posterolateral rotatory instability of the knee. *Am J Sports Med* 1983;11:199–207.
Loos WC, Fox JM, et al: Acute posterior cruciate ligament injuries. *Am J Sports Med* 1981;9:86–92.
Moore HA, Larson RL: Posterior cruciate ligament injuries. Results of early surgical repair. *Am J Sports Med* 1980;8:68–78.

Chronic PCL Repair

Clancy WG, Shelbourne KD, et al: Treatment of knee joint instability secondary to rupture of the posterior cruciate ligament. Report of new procedure. *J Bone Jt Surg,* 1983;65-A:310–322.
Fleming RE, Blatz DJ, McCarroll Jr: Posterior problems in the knee: Posterior cruciate insufficiency and posterolateral rotatory insufficiency. *Am J Sports Med* 1981;9:107–113.

18 Repair of Chronic Anterior Cruciate Ligament (ACL) Injuries

Clarence L. Shields, Jr.

General Considerations

The anterior cruciate ligament plays a major role in restraining the anterior displacement of the tibia on the femur. This is especially true in the last 15 to 20 degrees of extension.[1,2] Loss of this ligament may lead to a stretching of the secondary supporting structures on both the medial and the lateral sides of the knee. As a result, anteromedial and anterolateral rotational instability begins to develop. Usually, the menisci can restrain this development until they deteriorate with tears, which put the patient well on the road to degenerative changes in the joint. At this point, the patient experiences incapacitating symptoms of pain and feelings of definite instability when making deceleration turns.

The diagnosis of anterior cruciate ligament instability can be gauged as mild (+1), moderate (+2), or severe (+3). Several specific tests can be used. Straight anterior instability can be determined by the anterior drawer test in neutral rotation and by the Lachman test. Anterolateral instability can be diagnosed by either a positive jerk test or by a pivot shift. Anteromedial instability is determined by a positive anterior drawer test with 90 degrees of knee flexion and the foot in external rotation of 15 degrees.[3]

The natural history of the anterior cruciate deficient knee that remains untreated is well documented in the literature.[4] A plan of treatment can be individualized according to the following criteria: (1) the amount of instability; (2) the amount of degenerative arthritis; (3) the patient's age and activity; (4) the extent of meniscal injuries.

Treat patients who have mild instability with a rehabilitation program, provided the medial and lateral menisci are normal. Place individuals who are over the age of 45 years and have significant degenerative arthritis and sedentary life styles also on exercise programs. Put emphasis on hamstring exercises, starting isometrically and progressing to concentric and eccentric contractions. As strength improves, add Slocum and reverse Slocum exercises, since these exercises have been shown to decrease anterior subluxation of the tibia on the femur.[3,7] In the last phase of rehabilitation, once the hamstrings have become dominant, add quadriceps-strengthening exercises. To determine the conclusion of rehabilitation and to outline a maintenance program to follow, use a Cybex strength-and-power test. (For a complete discussion of this protocol, see Chap. 23.)

If the semilunar cartilages are damaged, perform a partial meniscectomy as well as a pes anserinus transfer and an iliotibial band transfer.[9,10] Studies show that either procedure alone will not withstand the stresses of continued athletic activity.[8,11] Moderate rotational instability requires the same procedures, with or without a mensicectomy. Patients with severe instability require the addition of an intra-articular patellar tendon substitution for the anterior cruciate ligament.[13] Also, patients who have moderate instability and are hyperelastic require the addition of the patellar tendon transfer. Contraindications to any of these operative procedures include the following: chondromalacia, Grade IV that involves either compartment of the knee joint, whether medial, lateral, or patellofemoral; a greater than 20-degree loss of motion in either flexion or extension since postoperative immobilization may increase the motion loss.

The surgical technique for the three procedures used to treat chronic anterior instability—pes anserinus transfer, Ellison procedure, and intra-articular patellar tendon transfer—will be described separately. However, surgically, the pes and Ellison are combined routinely, and the patellar tendon graft is added as needed.

Pes Anserinus Transfer

Surgical Procedure or Techniques

Place the patient in a supine position with a small bolster under the knee to produce approximately 30 degrees of knee flexion. Make an incision from the medial femoral epicondyle to slightly below the tibial tubercle (Fig. 18-1). Next, dissect the subcutaneous tissue with scissors up to the posteromedial aspect of the tibia. Take care to preserve the infrapatellar branch of the saphenous nerve. Mobilize the nerve enough to allow the pes tendons to be transferred beneath it.

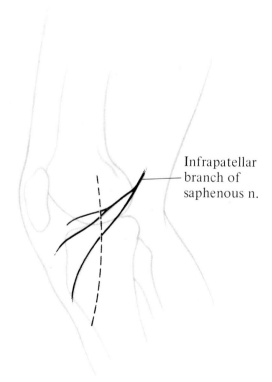

Infrapatellar branch of saphenous n.

FIGURE 18-1

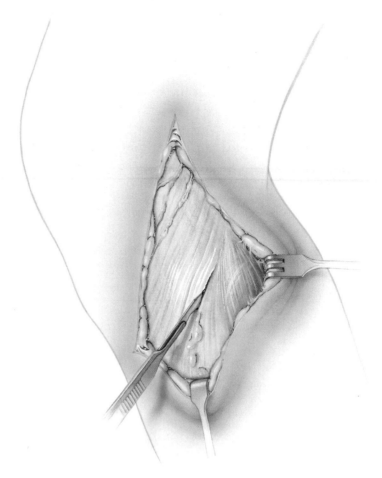

FIGURE 18-2

Identify the inferior border of the tendon at the junction of the muscle fibers of the medial gastrocnemius (Fig. 18-2). Sharply dissect this interval anteriorly toward the tibial crest and free the tendon from its periosteal attachment. Be sure not to cut the superficial medial collateral ligament anteriorly as the pes tendons are elevated from the tibia. Carry the anterior limb of the dissection no more than 1 cm below the superior border of the pes. Place a small Kocher's clamp on the inferior border and pull it anteriorly to expose more of the tendon.

Using scissors, separate carefully the tendon fibers from the fat over the main saphenous nerve and allow the fat to drop posteriorly, thus protecting the nerve. Continue the dissection proximally until the semimembranosis tendon attachment at the posterior medial tibia is felt (Fig. 18-3). Move the knee into more flexion, pull the pes tendons anteriorly, and reflect them so that their inferior borders are now superior.

Now, check the infrapatellar branch of the saphenous nerve to make sure that the transferred tendon does not bind or pinch this nerve before you begin suturing. Use #0 Vicryl on a round needle to avoid lacerations of the tendons. While maintaining traction, suture the anterior border into the periosteum adjacent to the patellar tendon. This maneuver will avoid patellar tendinitis later as the patient begins to generate internal rotational strength of the pes. Suture the upper border of the transferred tendon into the periosteum of the metaphyseal flair of the tibia, but avoid placing sutures into the superficial medial collateral ligament (Fig. 18-4). Otherwise, the patient will later experience a painful bursitis when the ligament excursion from anterior to posterior is prohibited.

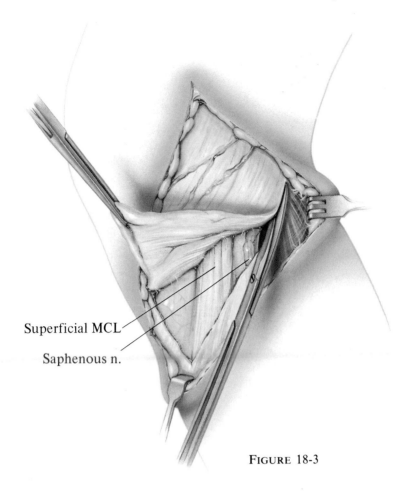

Superficial MCL

Saphenous n.

FIGURE 18-3

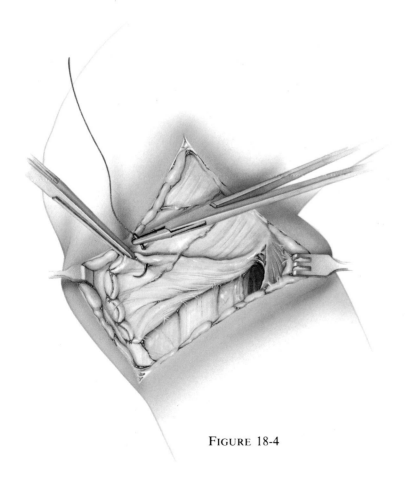

FIGURE 18-4

137

Finally, irrigate the wound with Garamycin solution and place a ⅛-inch Reliavac drain under the subcutaneous tissue to exit percutaneously above the patella in order to prevent an accumulation of postoperative wound hematoma. Close the subcutaneous tissue with #3-0 Dexon and the skin with #4-0 subcuticular nylon; apply Steri-strips.

The pes anserinus transfer is most often utilized in combination with the Ellison procedure for a moderate degree of anteromedial and anterolateral rotational instability of the knee. Occasionally, in severe medial collateral ligament injuries where there is a large amount of shredding of the medial capsule and collateral ligament, the pes transfer is added to the medial collateral ligament repair to reinforce the medial side. In this case, the pes transfer must be performed *after* the medial collateral ligament repair.

Ellison Procedure

Surgical Procedure and Techniques

Utilizing a thigh support, place the patient in the supine position with approximately 40 degrees of knee flexion. Make the lateral skin incision at least 3 cm anteriorly away from the medial skin incision. This will decrease the chances of a narrow skin bridge that might develop necrosis. Start the skin incision at the lateral femoral epicondyle, which is readily palpable, and extend it to Gerdy's tubercle on the anterolateral aspect of the tibial plateau (Fig. 18-5).

After dissecting the subcutaneous tissue, you can readily identify the anterolateral capsule and iliotibial band. At this point, take a sponge and wipe the fat globules off of the iliotibial band. This maneuver will allow identification of the superior portion of the iliotibial band adjacent to the anterolateral capsular fibers, which are slightly above and come in at a different angle from the iliotibial band (Fig. 18-6).

Sharply outline a 1.5-cm strip from Gerdy's tubercle and extend it towards the lateral femoral epicondyle. Osteotomize the iliotibial band, including approximately a 1.5-cm piece of bone from Gerdy's tubercle. Then, dissect the band superiorly, following the fibers with a slightly wider base. The base of the transfer should be approximately 2 cm wide and should be dissected proximal to the fibular collateral ligament by at least 1.5 cm.

The next step is to make a bony trough so that the bone fragment may be countersunk and advanced 1.5 cm anteriorly beneath the patellar tendon. Accomplish this maneuver with a small rongeur (Fig. 18-7). Now, change

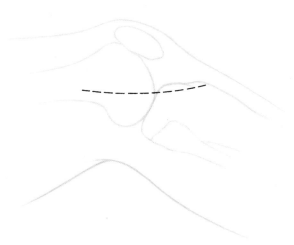

FIGURE 18-5

138

Iliotibial band   Patellar tendon

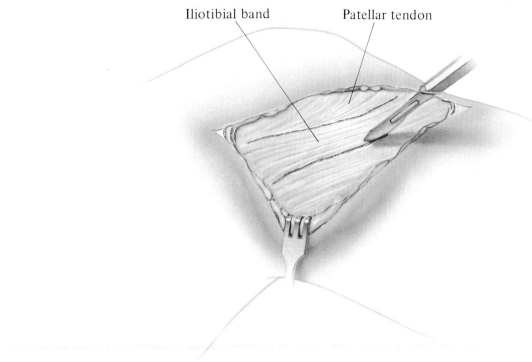

FIGURE 18-6

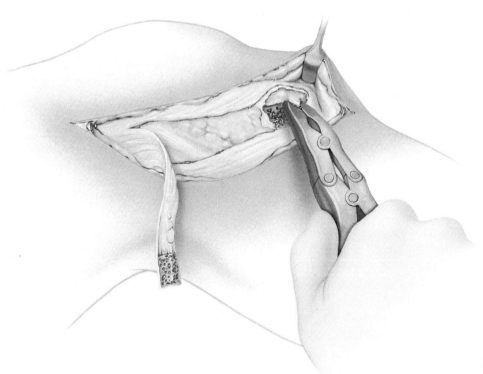

FIGURE 18-7

the position of the knee from 40 degrees to 90 degrees of flexion in order to palpate the fibular collateral ligament. Once it has been palpated, use a #15 blade to make an anterior and posterior cut on either side of the ligament.

Pass a large curved instrument beneath the fibular collateral ligament and dissect the area behind the ligament free from the synovium. At this point, open the joint and inspect it for changes in the articular cartilage and for meniscal damage. If necessary, do a partial meniscectomy under direct vision by placing the foot in the figure-of-four position and by applying varus stress to open the lateral compartment (Fig. 18-8). Close the synovium after the meniscectomy with #3–0 Dexon.

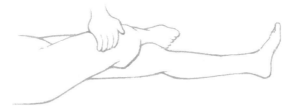

FIGURE 18-8. The figure-4 position.

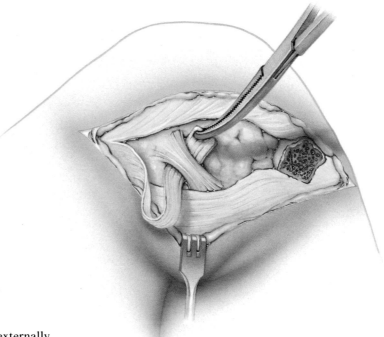

FIGURE 18-9. Tibia is rotated externally.

In order to pass the iliotibial band freely beneath the fibular collateral ligament, flex the knee more than 90 degrees while keeping the foot on the table. This relaxes the ligament and allows the transfer to be passed beneath it. As the transfer is passed, a gentle rocking motion in the direction of the fibular collateral ligament fibers is helpful (Fig. 18-9). Make sure that the transfer is near the femoral attachment of the ligament.

If a patellar tendon transfer is done at the same procedure, be certain to tie the sutures down at the femoral attachment of the intermuscular septum while keeping the knee in approximately 30 degrees of flexion *prior* to moving the transfer beneath the fibular collateral ligament. Place the small retractors anteriorly beneath the patellar tendon and test the bone block in its new bed to make sure that it fits adequately. It should be flush with the anterior surface of the tibia. Hold the foot in external rotation during this procedure of the operation to insure the advancement of the transfer. Use an orthopedic bone-cutting needle with #1 Ethibond suture to sew the transfer down in its new site.

During this portion of the operation, it may be necessary to extend the knee, but not beyond 40 degrees if a patellar tendon transfer is done at the same procedure. Place two sutures in position for tying them down, return the knee back into flexion, and hold the foot in external rotation while tying the sutures. Place two additional sutures in the most proximal portion of the bone block and into the periosteum of the tibia (Fig. 18-10).

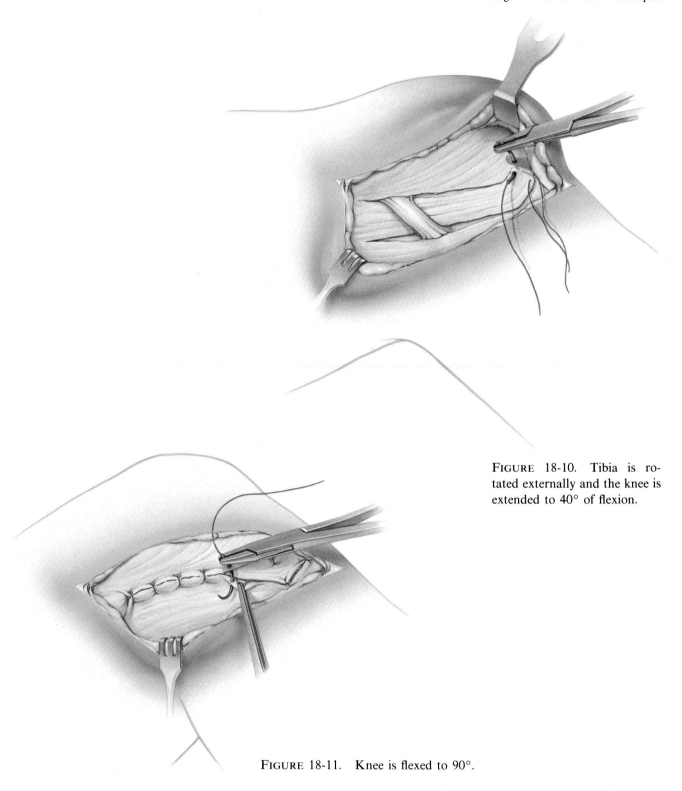

FIGURE 18-10. Tibia is rotated externally and the knee is extended to 40° of flexion.

FIGURE 18-11. Knee is flexed to 90°.

Utilize #0 Vicryl on a tapered needle for the capsular repair, since this tissue is thinner and a cutting needle may tear it. To bring the inferior limb of the capsule up towards the superior limb, use Vicryl. Flexion of the knee to 90 degrees or more will allow the capsular repair to be easily accomplished (Fig. 18-11). After the repair of the capsule is completed, extend the knee to 45 degrees gradually, making sure the sutures do not pull out. Close the subcutaneous tissue with #3–0 Dexon and the skin with #4–0 subcuticular nylon reinforced with Steri-strips. Use a Reliavac drain in the subcutaneous tissue to decrease the chances of a postoperative wound hematoma.

141

Remember that the Ellison procedure, which is utilized only in combination with other procedures such as pes anserinus transfer or patellar tendon graft, is the final procedure to be completed prior to closure of the capsule; for the knee position cannot be changed after the capsular incision is closed laterally.

Intra-Articular Patellar Tendon Transfer

Surgical Procedure and Techniques

Place the patient in a supine position with a small knee bolster to allow 40 degrees of knee flexion. Make a modified medial parapatellar incision from approximately 1 cm above the superior pole and extend it towards the tibial tubercle (Fig. 18-12). Undermine the subcutaneous tissue to expose the entire patella and the lateral border of its tendon, including the posteromedial corner. Usually, the infrapatellar branch of the saphenous nerve is sacrificed. Next, open the prepatellar bursa and tendon sheath longitudinally down the middle and preserve them both for closure. Then, dissect the subcutaneous tissue medially and laterally to the borders of the patellar tendon. After sharply outlining a 1 cm central strip of the patellar bone and tendon, try to preserve a 5 mm stump of quadriceps tendon proximally to serve as a handle.

Use an oscillating saw to cut a central strip of bone which is 5 mm thick and detach the patellar cortex from the superior pole distally with a curved osteotome. Take care to remove the inferior pole of the patella and tendon as a unit. Sharp dissection with a #15 blade is useful to complete the removal of the central strip of patellar tendon (Fig. 18-13).

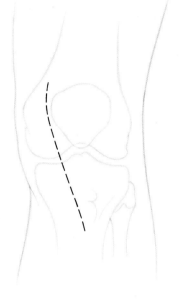

FIGURE 18-12

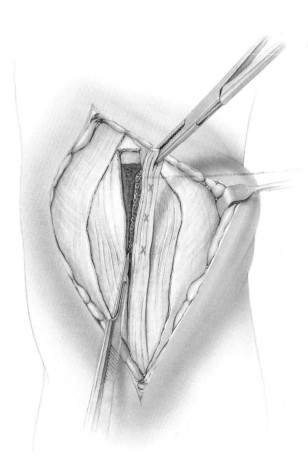

FIGURE 18-13. The three X's represent sites for drill holes.

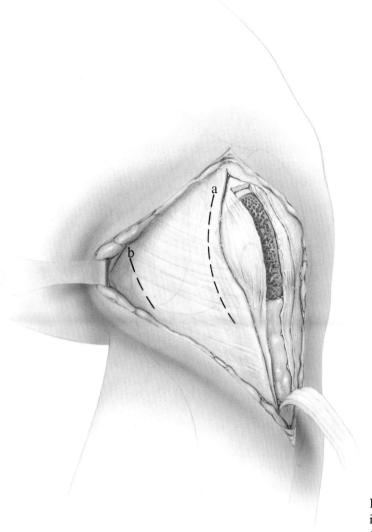

FIGURE 18-14. Locations of incisions for joint arthrotomies (a, b).

The next step is to make three drill holes, approximately 1 cm apart, in the patellar bone with a $\frac{5}{64}$-inch drill point. The bone can be easily drilled if the graft is returned to its bed in the patella. Perform a median parapatellar arthrotomy and inspect the joint (Fig. 18-14a). Place a Doane knee retractor (Z retractor) over the fat pad and a Blount retractor along the medial collateral ligament. Probe the medial meniscus from its anterior horn to the middle one-third.

A posteromedial capsular incision is required to visualize adequately the posterior horn. By removing the bolster, you can flex the knee to 90 degrees and palpate the soft spot behind the medial collateral ligament. The superior limb of this incision would be slightly more posterior than the inferior limb and curved obliquely towards the posterior edge of the medial collateral ligament (Fig. 18-14b). This oblique incision allows for better exposure behind the medial collateral ligament. Take care to avoid cutting the medial collateral ligament and also the superior portion of the medial meniscus. Place a Senn retractor on the posterior edge of the medial collateral ligament and a Doane knee retractor (Z retractor) in the posterior capsule. If indicated, a partial medial meniscectomy can be performed under direct vision to avoid injury to the posterior cruciate ligament.

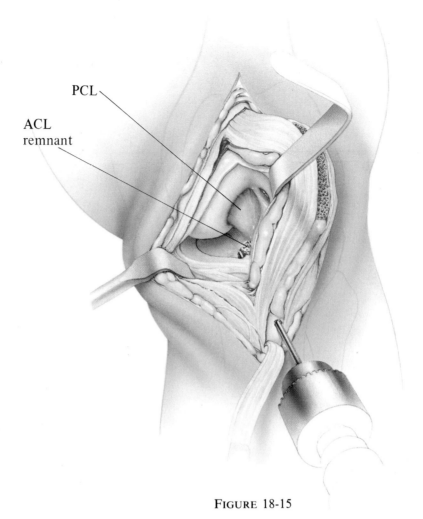

PCL

ACL
remnant

FIGURE 18-15

Now, move the retractors anteriorly and drill a $\frac{3}{32}$-inch smooth Steinmann pin from just above the attachment of the patellar tendon of the tibia and aim it to exit slightly anteromedial to the original tibial origin of the anterior cruciate ligament (Fig. 18-15). Use an 11-mm cannulated reamer to enlarge the hole, but take care not to lacerate the patellar tendon. Senn retractors are very useful in keeping the edges of the patellar tendon separate. Curette the tunnels and excise the soft tissue at the tibial articular surface exit.

Locate the femoral attachment of the anterior cruciate ligament. Start drilling a $\frac{3}{32}$-inch smooth pin approximately 1 cm posterior to the site on the lateral femoral condyle in the notch. This can readily be accomplished by placing the knee in the figure-of-four position (see Ellison procedure, above). The proper position of this hole is critical in restoring the posterolateral band of the anterior cruciate ligament.[13] Starting the pin in the notch assures that the location will be correct. Aim the pin at the lateral intermuscular septum, which can be readily palpated through the skin, and advance it until it tents the skin laterally.

Make a skin incision from Gerdy's tubercle on the tibia to just proximal to the pin. Then, dissect the subcutaneous tissue to expose the iliotibial band. Outline a 1-cm strip, osteotomize it with a piece of bone from Gerdy's tubercle, and retract the tissue proximal to the pin. This iliotibial band transfer will be longer than the routine Ellison procedure since the septum is more proximal on the femur. With an 11-mm cannulated reamer, drill over the pin from

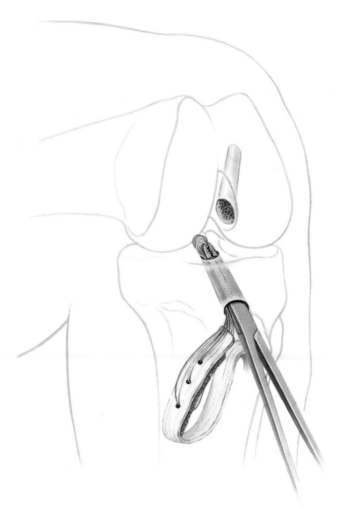

FIGURE 18-16

the lateral cortex towards the notch. Curette the hole and excise the soft tissue from the opening on the intra-articular side. A notchplasty is routinely done with a small osteotome to remove any osteophytes.

Place a tricolor-coated #1 Ethibond suture in each hole of the patellar bone graft and bring the proximal suture out through the end of the quadriceps tendon. Remove the needles and pass the sutures through the tibial hole with a straight hemostat and retrieve them in the joint (Fig. 18-16). Use a small forceps to maneuver the bone block within the joint. If the transfer does not slide freely in the hole, it should be removed, and both holes should be enlarged.

In passing the transfer, apply the major share of tension to the proximal suture, which is a different color. Thread the Richards' ligature passer from the lateral cortex into the joint and pull all three sutures through the femoral hole (Fig. 18-17). If a Richards' ligature passer is not available, an O'Donoghue suture passer, with a suture tied in a loop at the end, will catch all three ligatures.

While your assistant pulls on the proximal suture, maneuver the bone fragment into the tunnel. Then, while tension is being applied to the transfer, range the knee from extension to 40 degrees of flexion, and test the joint for anterior stability. The bone fragment must remain in the femoral tunnel. If this bone protrudes intra-articularly, osteotomize the graft from the tibial tubercle and advance it proximally as a free graft. In a similar fashion, drill the tibial attachment bone fragment. When a free graft must be utilized,

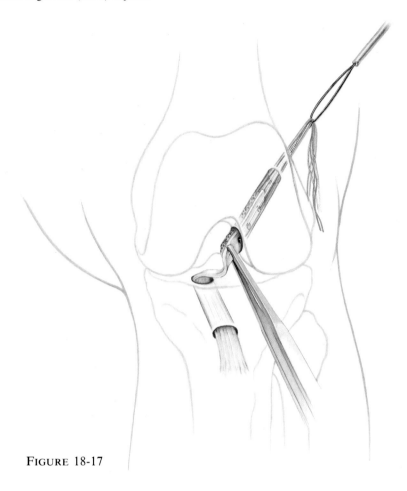

FIGURE 18-17

suture the femoral attachment to the intermuscular septum but adjust the final tension on the graft at the tibial end.

Now, open the lateral joint along the capsular incision and accomplish a partial meniscectomy. Also, prepare the bony trough for advancement of the iliotibial band under the patellar tendon. Dissect the fibular collateral ligament to allow passage of the iliotibial band beneath it.

Close the posteromedial capsule and perform the pes anserinus transfer prior to tying down the anterior cruciate ligament reconstruction. The tourniquet time should be checked; if it has exceeded 90 minutes, it should be released. The remainder of the procedure is performed without the tourniquet.

Thread a small curved free needle on one of the proximal Ethibond sutures and fasten it into the lateral intermuscular septum. While tying this one, have the assistant apply tension to the other sutures. After all three are sutured to the septum (Fig. 18-18), close the lateral synovium with #3–0 Dexon. Now, complete the Ellison procedure and close the capsule with #0 Vicryl on a tapered needle.

Through the anteromedial capsular incision, tack a distally based flap of synovium and fat pad around the graft with #4–0 Vicryl suture. Irrigate the joint with Garamycin solution; and if the patellar tendon has had to be advanced as a free graft, suture the distal attachment down into the remaining patellar tendon with #1 Ethibond and adjust the tension, as necessary, from the distal portion. Close the synovium with #3–0 Vicryl and #0 Vicryl for the capsule. Reapproximate the patellar tendon with #0 Vicryl, and close the bursa with #2–0 Vicryl over the patella. Insert a ⅛-inch Reliavac drain beneath the skin flap to exit above the knee. Finally, close the subcutaneous tissue with #3–0 Dexon and the skin with #4–0 clear Nylon in subcuticular

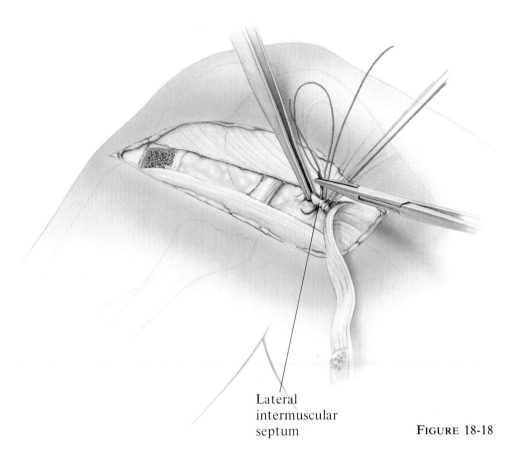

Lateral
intermuscular
septum

FIGURE 18-18

fashion. Reinforce the incision with Steri-strips and place the knee in anterior and posterior molded splints with 45 degrees of knee flexion and a neutral rotation of the tibia.

Postoperative Care and Rehabilitation

When the drainage from the knee, which has been immobilized at 45 degrees of flexion in anterior and posterior molded splints, becomes less than 50 cc in a 24- to 48-hour period, remove the drain from the subcutaneous tissue. Now, start the patient on isometric quadriceps, hamstrings, and calf exercises in the splint and allow the patient to ambulate, nonweightbearing, on crutches. At 2 weeks, change the splint and place the patient in a hinged cast or brace with a 45-degree extension stop. At this point, begin full weightbearing as tolerated.[12] The patient will be immobilized for 6 weeks.

At 6 weeks, remove the patient's cast and place the knee in a temporary brace, such as a Don Joy System II short-phase. Set the brace at a 40-degree extension stop and start the patient who will be maintained in the brace for the next 3 months, on physical therapy. Instruct the patient on how to sleep in the brace for the first 3 weeks. This brace, which will accommodate a large increase in thigh circumference, can be utilized until the patient reaches the last phase of rehabilitation. At that point, when the thigh atrophy is less than 1 cm, make a mold for the derotational brace that will be utilized for 1 full year postsurgery.

When the pes anserinus transfer and Ellison procedures are utilized without a patellar tendon graft, the knee can be brought out into extension before 3

147

months, since there is no revascularization of any intra-articular structure.[14,15] (Maintain the patient in the physical therapy program outlined under anterior cruciate instability in Chap. 23.)

References

Pes Anserinus Transfer

1. Henning CE, Lynch MA: An in vivo strain gauge study of the anterior cruciate ligament. Presented at the annual meeting of the International Society for the Knee. Lyon, France, April 1979.
2. Cabaud HE: Biomechanics of the anterior cruciate ligament. *Clin Orthop* 1983;172:26–31.
3. Slocum DB, Larson RL: Rotatory instability of the knee, its pathogenesis and a clinical test to demonstrate its presence. *J Bone Jt Surg* 1968;50-A:211–225.
4. McDaniel WJ Jr, Dameron TB Jr: Untreated ruptures of the anterior cruciate ligament. A follow-up study, *J Bone Jt Surg* 1980;62-A:696–705.
5. Giove TP, Miller SJ, et al: Non-operative treatment of the torn anterior cruciate ligament. *J Bone Jt Surg.* 1983;65-A:184–192.
6. Paulos L, Noyes FR, et al: Knee rehabilitation after anterior cruciate ligament reconstruction and repair. *Am J Sports Med* 1981;9:140–149.
7. Noyes FR, Sonstegard DA: Biochemical function of the pes anserinus at the knee and the effect of its transplantation. *J Bone Jt Surg* 1973;55-A:1225–1241.
8. Beyer AH, Shields CL, et al: Extra-articular reconstruction of the anterior cruciate ligament. Presented at the annual meeting of the American Orthopaedic Society for Sports Medicine. Williamsburg, VA, July 1983.

Ellison Procedure

9. Ellison, AE: Distal iliotibial-band transfer for anterolateral rotatory instability of the knee. *J Bone Jt Surg,* 1979;61-A:330–337.
10. Losee RE, Johnson TR, Southwick WO: Anterior subluxation of the lateral tibial plateau, a diagnostic test and operative repair. *J Bone Jt Surg* 1978;60-A:1015–1030.
11. MacIntosh DL, Darby TA: Lateral subluxation reconstruction. *J Bone Jt Surg* 1976;58B:142.

Intra-Articular Patellar Tendon Transfer

12. Haggmark TN, Eriksson E: Cylinder or mobile cast brace after knee ligament surgery. A clinical analysis and morphologic and enzymatic studies of changes in the quadriceps muscle. *Am J Sports Med* 1979;7:48–56.
13. Clancy WG, Jr., Nelson DA, et al: Anterior cruciate ligament reconstruction using one-third of the patellar ligament, augmented by extra-articular tendon transfer. *J Bone Jt Surg* 1982;64-A:352–359.
14. Cabaud HE, Rodkey WG, et al: Experimental studies of acute anterior cruciate ligament injury and repair. *Am J Sports Med* 1979;7:18–22.
15. Cabaud HE, Feagin JA, et al: Acute anterior cruciate ligament injury and augmented repair. Experimental studies. *Am J Sports Med* 1980;8:395–401.

Additional Reading

Bassett GS, Fleming BW: The Lenox Hill Brace in anterolateral rotatory instability. *Am J Sports Med* 1983;11:345–348.

Fleming RE, Blatz DJ, McCarroll JR: Lateral reconstruction for anterolateral rotatory instability of the knee. *Am J Sports Med* 1983;11:303–307.

Fried JA, Bergfeld JA, et al: Anterior cruciate reconstruction using the Jones-Ellison Procedure. *J Bone Jt Surg.* 1985;67-A:1029–1033.

Hanks GA, Joyner DM, Kalenak A: Anterolateral rotatory instability of the knee: An analysis of the Ellison procedure. *Am J Sports Med* 1981;9:225–232.

Hester JT, Falkel JE; Isokinetic evaluation of tibial rotation: Assessment of a stabilization technique. *J Orthop Sports Phys Ther* 1984;1:46–51.

Ritter MA, Leaming ES, McCarroll Jr: Preliminary report of the Jones, Ellison, Slocum (JES) repair for symptomatic anterior cruciate deficient knee. *Am J Sports Med* 1983;11:89–94.

Simonet WT, Sim FH: Repair and reconstruction of rotatory instability of the knee. *Am J Sports Med* 1984;12:89–97.

Teitge RA, Indelicato PA, et al: Iliotibial band transfer for anterolateral rotatory instability of the knee: Summary of 54 cases. *Am J Sports Med* 1980;8:223–227.

Univerferth LJ, Bagenstose JE: Extra-articular reconstructive surgery for combined anterolateral anteromedial rotatory instability. *Am J Sports Med* 1979;7:34–39.

Ankle IV

19 Arthroscopy

Lewis A. Yocum

General Considerations

Arthroscopy of the ankle can be easily carried out. But, unlike the knee, the ankle is less forgiving. A thorough knowledge of the anatomy is thus essential before beginning. Familiarity with the use of the spinal needle for joint distention and triangulation is also beneficial. We find it helpful to use a marking pen to delineate important landmarks that may become distorted as arthroscopy proceeds. The important ones to remember are the medial and lateral malleoli and the extensor tendons.

Surgical Procedure and Techniques

The procedure can be done under a local, regional, or general anesthetic. Place the patient in a supine position on the operating table and apply a pneumatic cuff to the thigh. After effective anesthesia is instituted, test the extremity for ligamentous stability. Do sterile preparation and drape the leg free.

By dorsiflexing and plantarflexing the foot, the joint can be identified. The primary portals are an anteromedial and anterolateral approach. Inject local anesthetic with a 21-guage needle at the portal sites. The anterolateral portal is at the joint level just lateral to the extensor digitorum longus tendon. (Fig. 19–1). The anteromedial portal is just medial to the anterior tibial tendon (Fig. 19–1). The use of a small arthroscopy (a 2.2-mm sleeve) may aid in viewing the entire joint (Fig. 19–2); however, the standard arthroscope often facilitates inspection posteriorly in the ankle joint.

If access to the posterior aspect of the ankle is less than optimal, a postero-lateral portal can be used (Fig. 19–3). Insert a spinal needle just lateral to the Achilles tendon.

Continuous irrigation is difficult and generally not necessary. Local distention can be carried out through the scope or with a syringe and a 16-gauge needle inserted at another site. The use of the spinal needle for triangulation aids in the insertion of operative instruments.

152

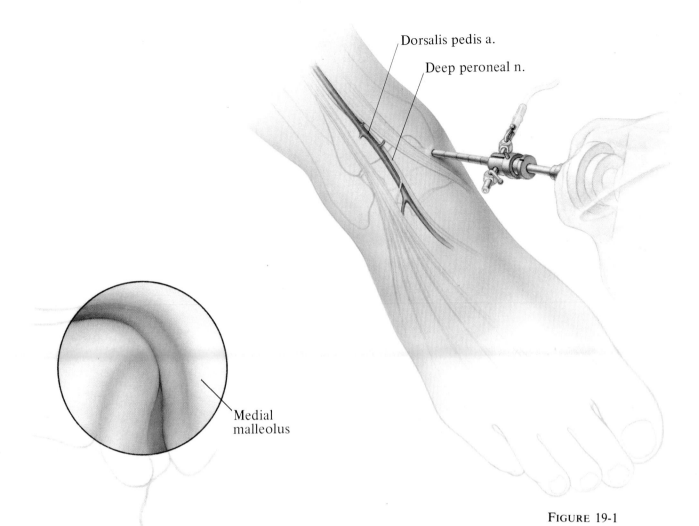

Dorsalis pedis a.

Deep peroneal n.

Medial malleolus

FIGURE 19-1

FIGURE 19-2. Medial gutter.

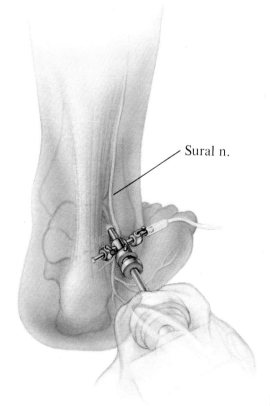

Sural n.

FIGURE 19-3

153

References

1. Johnson, LL: *Diagnostic and Surgical Arthroscopy, the Knee and Other Joints.* St. Louis, Mosby, 1981, pp 412–419.
2. Drez D, Guhl JF, Gollehon DL: Ankle arthroscopy: Technique and indications. *Clin Sports Med* 1982;1:35–45.

Additional Reading

Heller AJ, Vogler HW: Ankle joint arthroscopy. *J Foot Surg* 1982;21:23–29.

Parisien JS, Shereff JM: The role of arthroscopy in diagnosis and treatment of disorders of the ankle. *Foot Ankle* 1981;2:144–149.

Pritsch M, Horoshovski H, Farine I: Ankle arthroscopy. *Clin Orthop* 1984;184:137–140.

Repair of Achilles Tendon Injuries

20

Clarence L. Shields, Jr.

Tendinitis and Partial Rupture Repair

General Considerations

Generally, inflammatory conditions involving the Achilles tendon develop gradually. Patients usually complain of pain and a limp after strenuous exercise. The precipitating events are frequently speed training or interval workouts. The deceleration or cutting maneuver that occurs when a runner rapidly changes direction increases the pain. Repeated microtrauma to the fibers causes tendon edema and tissue inflammation. When enough fibers are affected, symptoms become evident. The potential for athletes to sustain such microtrauma, however, is great. In jogging, for example, there are approximately 1,500 heel strikes per mile, with the triceps surae contracting on each strike.

In patients with acute tendinitis, gentle palpation of the tendon as the ankle moves from plantarflexion to dorsiflexion will reveal crepitation in 50 percent of the patients.[1] There may be tenderness anywhere along the tendon from the muscle belly to the os calcis attachment. In patients over the age of 30 years, a lateral X-ray should be taken to look for tendon calcification or a heel spur anterior to the tendon. Either of these findings may be responsible for a chronic problem.

Two weeks of rest are required for patients with acute symptoms. We also recommend the use of nonsteroidal anti-inflammatory drugs and a $5/16$-inch heel lift in the shoe. As the symptoms decrease, a stretching and strengthening program should begin. Before engaging in physical activity, the patient should use heat; afterwards, ice. In patients with excessive heel varus, orthotic devices may be required.

In cases of Achilles tendinitis that resist the usual treatment, the affected leg should be placed in a short leg walking cast with the foot in equinus for 3 weeks. In chronic cases, the tendon becomes thickened and indurated as well as painful. Those patients whose symptoms persist after 6 months of conservative therapy may require the resection of the tendon sheath or of an area of necrotic tendon and the reconstruction with a fascial graft. Occasionally, the tendon may be irritated by a prominent superior tuberosity of the os calcis.[1]

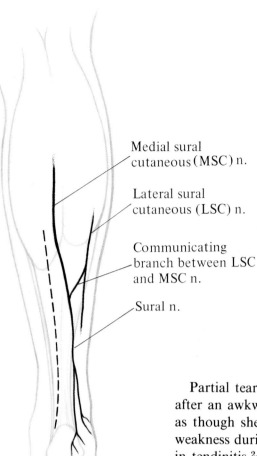

Medial sural
cutaneous (MSC) n.

Lateral sural
cutaneous (LSC) n.

Communicating
branch between LSC
and MSC n.

Sural n.

FIGURE 20-1

Partial tears of the Achilles tendon begin with an acute tearing sensation after an awkward step or fall. The patient may hear an audible snap or feel as though she were struck with a tennis ball and then experience pain and weakness during push-off. This contrasts with the gradual onset of symptoms in tendinitis.[2,3] A partial rupture of the tendon can be distinguished from a complete rupture by a negative Thompson test, in which the manual compression of the calf will cause plantarflexion of the foot. This occurs because most of the tendon fibers remain intact.[4] A partially torn tendon initially has a localized tender area, but after 2 weeks it adheres to the sheath and becomes thickened and indurated. Histological studies of the tendon usually show chronically inflamed devitalized tissue. Chronic partial ruptures require the same treatment as chronic tendinitis.

Surgical Procedure and Techniques

Anesthetize the patient in the supine position, then turn him prone. To allow for chest expansion, place rolled towels or bolsters longitudinally under the patient from the iliac spine up to the anterior shoulder. In males, be sure to check the position of the genitalia.

We prefer a skin incision on the medial side of the tendon in order to avoid injury to the sural nerve. Extend the incision from the medial calf down to the heel (Fig. 20–1). In the proximal portion of the wound, the medial cutaneous nerve of the calf should be protected; in the distal portion, the incision should stay above the level of the shoe counter. Dissect the subcutaneous tissue medially and laterally to expose the tendon sheath. After opening the tendon sheath, excise all areas of necrosis. Usually, this excising will not involve the entire width of the tendon; therefore the fascial graft will be narrower than the one used for complete rupture (Fig. 20–2). Also, since part of the tendon is intact, the defect cannot be sutured end to end. The graft will bridge this gap in the tendon when it is sutured to the intact tendon with #0 Vicryl on a tapered needle (Fig. 20–3). Close the fascial donor site with #0 Vicryl. Place the patient in a short leg cast with gravity equinus position of the foot.

156

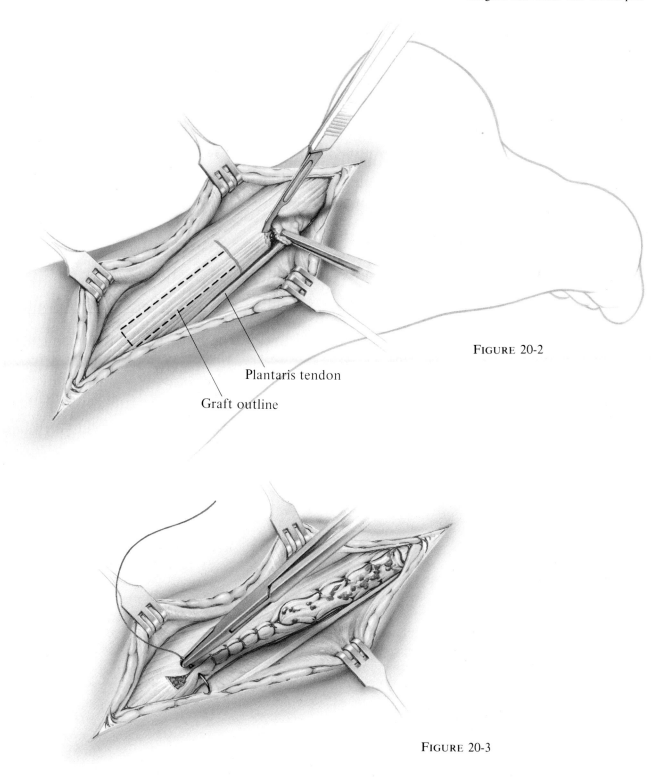

Plantaris tendon

Graft outline

FIGURE 20-2

FIGURE 20-3

In the patient with a prominent os calcis beak, the distal limb of the incision may be extended towards the heel. If the beak is excised, take care to protect the tendon from the osteotome (Fig. 20–4). Use the appropriate size of the Hoke osteotome and smooth the bed with a nasal rasp to minimize any prominence. Reapproximate the tendon sheath with #2–0 and #3–0 Dexon, and close the subcutaneous tissue with #3–0 Dexon. Close the skin with #4–0 subcuticular nylon and reinforce it with Steri-strips.

157

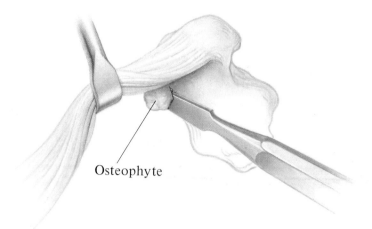

Osteophyte

FIGURE 20-4

Postoperative Recovery and Rehabilitation

Immobilize the patient with a partial rupture repair for 3 weeks while only 2 weeks with os calcis beak resection. Both injuries are placed in a short leg cast with gravity equinus position of the foot. The rehabilitation program is the same for those patients who undergo either a partial or a complete rupture repair of the Achilles tendon (Chap. 23), including the wearing of a half-inch heel lift for 3 months.

Complete Rupture Repair

General Considerations

Complete ruptures of the Achilles tendon usually occur in athletes who play basketball, volleyball, or similar sports in which a great deal of jumping is involved. The mechanism of injury is violent dorsiflexion of the foot, either while extending the knee or while pushing off with the weightbearing foot plantarflexed. When the calf muscles are strongly contracted, a sudden violent force to the foot will often lead to marked stretching of the muscle and tendon. At the time of such a rupture, the patient either hears or feels a snap in the calf, which is followed by immediate pain and weakness in the same area.[5]

Our studies reveal that patients who experience acute ruptures of the Achilles tendon fall into two categories: those who have had symptoms prior to the rupture, and those who have had no symptoms before the rupture.[6] The majority of patients fall into the second category. Also, the physical conditioning of a patient does not appear to influence the incidence of rupture. The usual site of the disruption is approximately 2 to 3 cm above the attachment to the os calcis. In the Thompson test, the patient's foot will not plantarflex when the calf muscle is squeezed because the tendon is not in continuity. Acute ruptures in the athlete should be repaired surgically.

Surgical Procedure and Techniques

The position of the patient and the incision location are the same as for a partial rupture (Fig. 20–1). In the proximal portion of the wound, the medial cutaneous nerve of the calf should be protected; in the distal portion, the incision should stay above the level of the shoe counter.

158

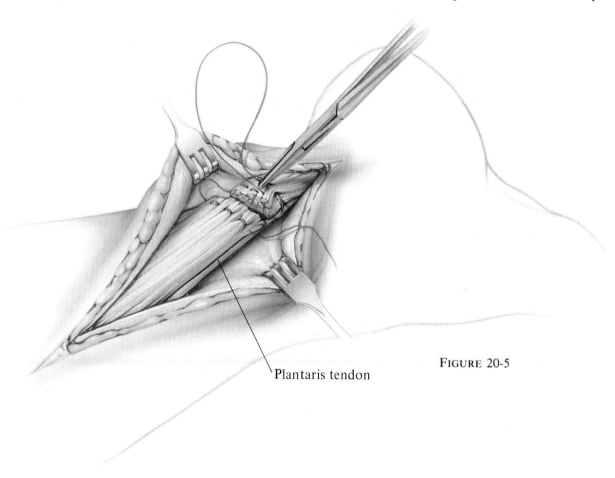

Plantaris tendon

FIGURE 20-5

Dissect the subcutaneous tissue medially and laterally to expose the blood-filled tendon sheath. Open it down the middle so that it can later be closed over the repair. Remove the clots from around the tendon ends and send some tissue to the lab for biopsy. The plantaris tendon is usually found to be intact. Use an atraumatic needle with #0 Polydek suture in a horizontal mattress fashion to approximate the ends with the foot in equinus (Fig. 20-5).

It is important to weave the sutures through the tendon fibers in each tendon stump. Mark the tendon 1.5 cm proximal to the suture line with methylene blue. After locating the base at the blue mark, outline a flap of the central portion of the gastrocnemius fascia and Achilles tendon. Mark the flap so it is long enough to go at least 1 cm distal to the suture line. Use a #15 knife blade to make a partial thickness flap that leaves enough tendon medially and laterally to close the defect (Fig. 20-6).

Suture the flap with #0 Vicryl on a tapered needle and wrap the flap around the tendon (Fig. 20-7). Also, close the defect in the fascia with #0 Vicryl. Close the tendon sheath with #00 Dexon proximally and #3-0 Dexon distally, since the sheath is thinner in the distal portion of the incision. Next, close the subcutaneous tissue with Dexon and the skin with 4-0 nylon in a subcuticular fashion reinforced with Steri-strips.

Place the patient in a short leg cast while in the prone position with the foot in gravity equinus. Then, turn the patient supine, but do not allow the knee to go into extension. Complete the cast by constructing a long leg cast with 45 degrees of knee flexion.

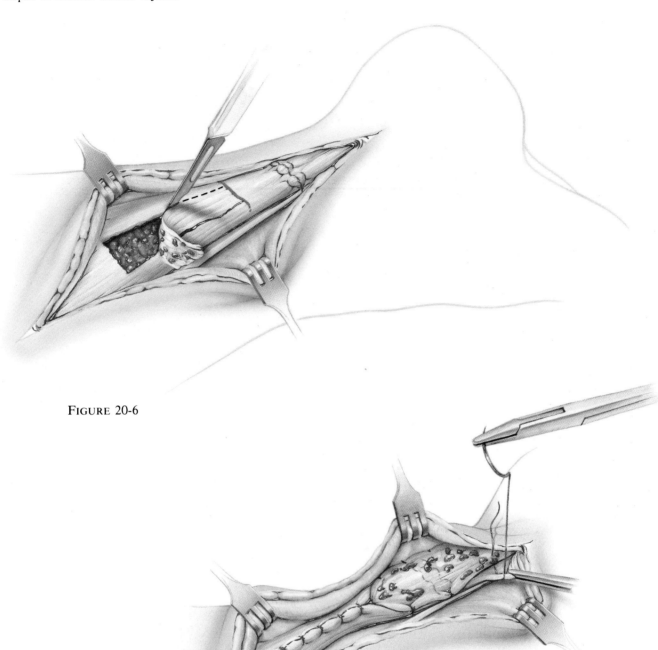

FIGURE 20-6

FIGURE 20-7

Postoperative Recovery and Rehabilitation

Immobilize the patient for 1 month in a long leg cast with the foot in equinus. At 1 month, place the patient in a short leg walking cast with the foot still in equinus. This casting will require a buildup of the heel to allow the patient to ambulate. This is followed by 6 months of wearing a half-inch heel lift on the involved leg. Initially, rehabilitation involves exercises for isometric plantarflexion.[7]

Following isometric exercises, the therapy advances to active resistive exercises, including rubberband exercises and toe raises as tolerated by the patient.

Add progressive resistive exercises with weights by instituting toe raises on either a shoulder-press machine or on a leg-press or isokinetic device (See Chap. 23). There is no stretching of the tendon for at least 3 months. Have the patient continue to work out after returning to athletics and continue to wear the heel lift for 6 months.

Cybex strength evaluations at 6 months, 9 months, and 12 months postoperatively show that calf muscle strength does not return to normal until at least 1 year after the repair of the tendon. Cybex isokinetic evaluations of repairs of the Achilles tendon show a 16.5 percent loss of plantarflexion strength and a 17.5 percent loss of plantarflexion power. Early repairs have smaller losses of strength and power than do late repairs. As many as 27 patients out of 33 have been able to return to their former level of sports activity.[5]

References

Tendinitis and Partial Rupture Repair

1. Leach RE, Wasilewski JS: Achilles tendinitis. *Am J Sports Med* 1981;9:93–98.
2. Skeoch, DU: Spontaneous partial subcutaneous ruptures of the tendo Achilles. Review of the literature and evaluation of 16 involved tendons. *Am J Sports Med* 1981;9:20–22.
3. Ljungqvist R: Subcutaneous partial rupture of the Achilles tendon. *Acta Orthop Scand* 1967 (suppl);113:1–86.
4. Thompson TC, Doherty JH: Spontaneous rupture of tendo Achilles. A new clinical diagnostic test. *J Trauma* 1962;2:126–129.

Complete Rupture Repair

5. Shields CL, Kerlan RK, Jobe FW et al: The Cybex II evaluation of surgically repaired Achilles tendon ruptures. *Am J Sports Med* 1978;6:369–372.
6. Fox JM, Blazina ME, Jobe FW, et al: Degeneration and rupture of the Achilles tendon. *Clin Orthop* 1975:221–224.
7. Shields CL: Achilles tendon injuries. *Phys Sports Med* 1982;10:77–84.

Additional Reading

Clement DB, Taunton JE, Smart GW: Achilles tendinitis and peritendinitis: Etiology and treatment. *Am J Sports Med* 1984;12:179–184.
Kuwada GT, Schuberth J: Evaluation of Achilles tendon reruptures *J Foot Surg* 1984;23:340–343.
Leach RE, Dilorio E, Harney RA: Pathologic hindfoot conditions in the athlete. *Clin Orthop* 1983;177:116–121.
Nistor L: Surgical and non-surgical treatment of Achilles tendon rupture. A prospective randomized study. *J Bone Jt Surg* 1981;63-B:394–399.
O'Brien T: The needle test for complete rupture of the Achilles tendon. *J Bone Jt Surg* 1984;66-A:1099–1101.

21 Repair of Chronic Lateral Ligament Injuries

Lewis A. Yocum

Brostrom Procedure for Reconstruction

General Considerations

The ideal of any ligament reconstruction is to attempt to restore the anatomy to its normal state before injury. In dealing with the lateral ligaments of the ankle, one would ideally like to be able to restore also their normal anatomic configuration. The Brostrom technique affords the surgeon the opportunity to attempt to restore the normal structures of the anterior talofibular and fibulocalcaneal ligaments.[1]

Surgical Procedure and Techniques

After an effective level of anesthesia is reached, place the patient in a lateral decubitus position with the affected extremity at a comfortable level for surgical procedure. Provide proper padding for all bony prominences as well as nerves on the dependent side. Prep the leg and drape it in the usual fashion. Use an Esmarch bandage to exsanguinate the extremity and a hemostatic cuff to provide a bloodfree field. Start a curvilinear skin incision just distal to the lateral malleolus and course it over the region of the sinus tarsi (Fig. 21–1). Carry dissection down through the subcutaneous tissue, where you will generally find fatty synovial tissue that is thickened and scarred.

Palpation of the anterior aspect of the talofibular region will generally reveal a "soft spot," which can be entered in order to expose the articular surfaces of the talus and fibula (Fig. 21–2). Blunt reflection with a curette and/or perosteal elevator will expose the anterior tibiofibular ligament; at this point, careful dissection distally will expose the anterior talofibular ligament.

A careful review of the anatomy of this region is important, since the anterior talofibular ligament is frequently bound in scar and occasionally calcified in part. Both proximal and distal ends of the ligament should be exposed. Defects occasionally occur in midsubstance. However, we have more commonly noted an avulsion from the anterior aspect of the fibula. This can occur with or without a piece of bone. Should a small fragment of bone be found in the ligament, dissect it sharply from the ligament. Exploration of the calcaneofibular ligament is essential.

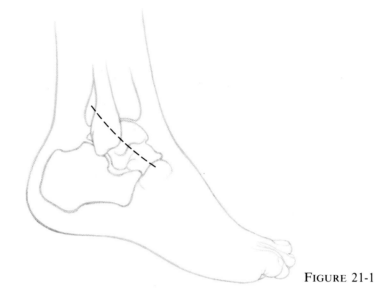

FIGURE 21-1

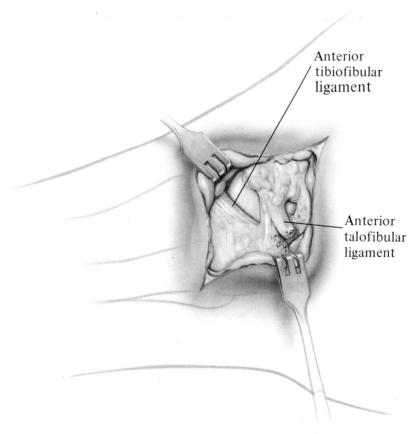

Anterior
tibiofibular
ligament

Anterior
talofibular
ligament

FIGURE 21-2

Opening the peroneal sheath will expose the ligament (Fig. 21–3), which is quite often intact. Although it may be stretched, its competency can be evaluated by forcing the heel into inversion. Should repair be necessary, suturing can be carried out at this time. For a midsubstance tear of the anterior talofibular ligament, hold the foot in a neutral position, freshen the end of the ligament, and carry out a primary end-to-end repair. Generally, a #2–0 nonabsorbable suture is used and reinforced with an absorbable suture. In the more common situation where the anterior talofibular ligament has been avulsed from the anterior aspect of the fibula, create a trough in the anterior

163

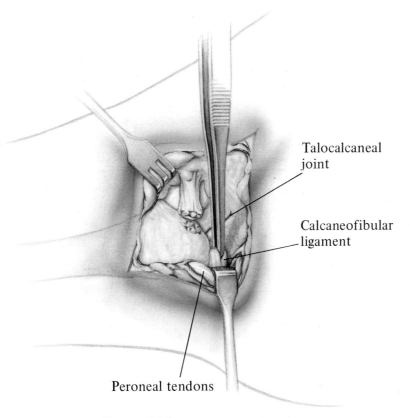

Talocalcaneal
joint

Calcaneofibular
ligament

Peroneal tendons

FIGURE 21-3

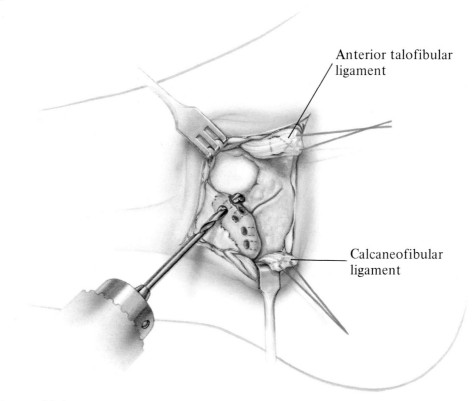

Anterior talofibular
ligament

Calcaneofibular
ligament

FIGURE 21-4

aspect of the fibula by using a small osteotome. Smooth the edges with a rongeur and then drill two holes with a $\frac{5}{16}$ drill bit just posterior to the fibular trough (Fig. 21–4). Place a Bunnell suture through the anterior talofibular ligament, draw the ligament to the fibula, and pass the sutures through

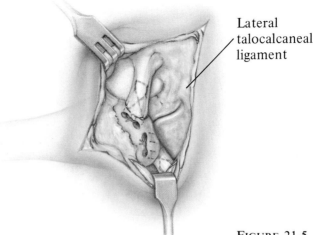

Lateral talocalcaneal ligament

FIGURE 21-5

the drill holes before securing the ligament to the fibula (Fig. 21–5). Again, take care to position the foot properly before securing sutures.

Occasionally, the remnants of the anterior talofibular ligament are too scant to permit a primary repair. In this case, a small strip of the lateral talocalcaneal ligament can be used to reinforce the anterior talofibular ligament. Irrigate the wound with Garamycin solution and check for hemostasis with Bovie electrocautery on identifiable vessels. If the peroneal sheath was opened for inspection, close it in an interrupted fashion with a #2–0 Vicryl suture.

Reapproximate subcutaneous tissues loosely with an absorbable suture, and close the skin with #4–0 clear nylon in a subcuticular fashion and reinforce with Steri-strips. Apply sterile dressing and place the patient in a well-padded posteromedial plaster splint.

Postoperative Recovery and Rehabilitation

Have the patient begin nonweight-bearing crutch ambulation on the first post-operative day. Inspect the patient's wound 2 weeks postoperatively, at which time change him to a short leg cast for an additional 3 weeks. At this point, remove the cast and have him continue using crutches for assistive ambulation. An ankle lacer is used for additional 4 weeks. Concurrently, start him on a range of motion and muscle-strengthening exercises (Chap. 23).

Chrisman-Snook Procedure for Reconstruction

General Considerations

In recent years, chronic lateral instability of the ankle has become more common and a better-recognized entity. Quite often, the physician confronts an athlete who has a history of repeated sprains that cause recurrent swelling as well as apprehension in performing athletic maneuvers. The discomfort may be isolated to the anterior talofibular ligament and the fibulocalcaneal ligament; or it may be more diffuse around the region of the sinus tarsi. Chronic synovitis of this area is a frequent accompaniment to lateral instability.

The surgical approach to the problem of chronic lateral instability is that of the Chrisman-Snook modification of the Elmslie tenodesis of the ankle.[2,3] This is especially true in individuals who present with extensive destruction of both the anterior talofibular and the fibulocalcaneal ligaments.

165

Surgical Procedure and Techniques

For most repairs, a general anesthetic is effective. Place the patient in a lateral decubitis position with the lateral aspect of the affected extremity at a comfortable level for the surgical procedures. Take care to provide proper support for the trunk as well as proper padding for any bony prominence on the dependent side. It is equally important to provide a relief area for the peroneal nerve and padding for the dependent ankle. Prep the affected extremity and drape it in the usual fashion. Wrap the leg with an Esmarch bandage to exsanguinate the extremity, and inflate a hemostatic cuff to approximately 100 mm above systolic pressure (generally 250 mm).

Open the surgical stockinette to expose the lateral aspect of the ankle and foot. Place the skin incision over the route of the peroneus brevis tendon in a "lazy S" fashion. This affords easier access to the lateral calcaneus. When making the incision, the foot is held in a neutral (i.e. a right angle) position. This will make postoperative closure and splinting easier. The incision course is along the posterior aspect of the fibula, curving anteriorly at the inferior tip of the lateral malleolus and extending distally to the base of the fifth metatarsal (Fig. 21–6). In making the initial incision, take care not to disturb the cutaneous nerves, and pay special attention to the sural nerve. Enlarge the operative field and reflect the anterior flap of skin over the lateral malleolus. In creating a flap, be sure that it is not too thin; otherwise, the risk of skin loss postoperatively will be greater.

Identify the peroneus brevis tendon and split it longitudinally from its muscle belly to the base of the fifth metatarsal (Fig. 21–7). Dorsiflexion and plantarflexion of the foot aids in division of the tendon as it passes beneath the lateral malleolus. Leave the superior retinacular pulley of the peroneal tendons at the level of the lateral malleolus intact. If it is necessary to incise the lower pulleys, take care to reconstruct these prior to closure. Detach the split peroneus brevis proximally, but leave it attached at the base of the fifth metatarsal.

Place a horizontal drill hole through the distal fibula at the level of the ankle mortise and course it from an anterior to posterior direction (Fig. 21–8). Generally, a ¼-inch drill bit is satisfactory for this task. Use a curette to enlarge the ends of the hole to allow free passage of the tendon graft. Use a small periosteal elevator to strip the soft tissue from the anterior talofibular ligament.

At this time, open the interval between the anterior talofibular ligament and the anterior tibiofibular ligament to explore the anterior aspect of the ankle. Now, pass the split peroneus brevis tendon from an anterior to a poste-

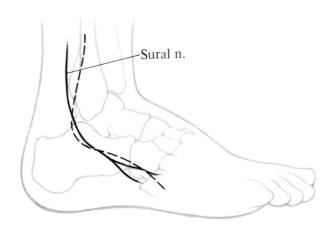

Sural n.

FIGURE 21-6

166

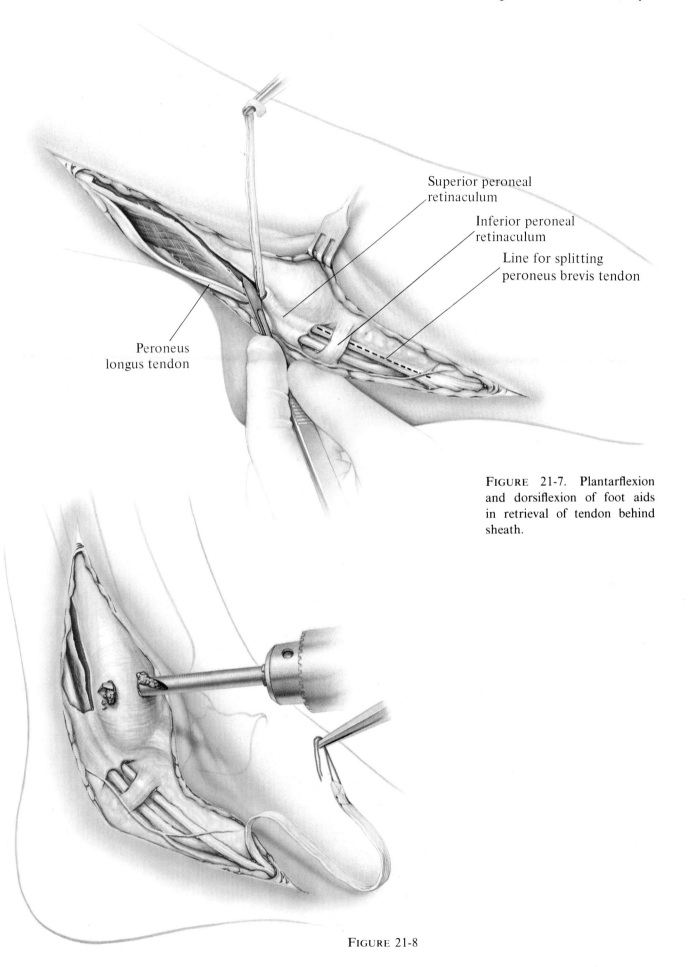

Superior peroneal
retinaculum

Inferior peroneal
retinaculum

Line for splitting
peroneus brevis tendon

Peroneus
longus tendon

FIGURE 21-7. Plantarflexion
and dorsiflexion of foot aids
in retrieval of tendon behind
sheath.

FIGURE 21-8

167

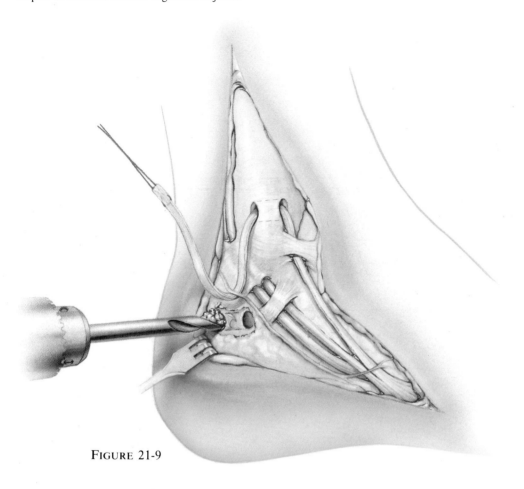

FIGURE 21-9

rior direction through the fibula, and then bring it distally coursing over the peroneus longus tendon but beneath the sural nerve—to the lateral border of the calcaneus. As opposed to the classical osteoperiosteal flaps, use a ¼-inch drill coursing in a posterior to an anterior direction to create a tunnel in the lateral aspect of the calcaneus distal to the tip of the lateral malleolus (Fig. 21–9). Curette the hole, then pass the tendon, coursing from a posterior to an anterior direction, through the calcaneal drill hole and bring it out to the base of the fifth metatarsal.

Now, hold the foot in a reduced posture, with the heel in a neutral to a slightly everted position and the foot at a right angle to the leg. Apply tension to the tendon graft, and place nonabsorbable sutures between the peroneus brevis graft and the anterior talofibular ligament. Draw the ligament snugly through the fibula, and place sutures through the periosteum at both the anterior and posterior aspects of the calcaneal tunnel. Then, suture the tendon in place to the base of the fifth metatarsal (Fig. 21–10). If the split tendon is too short, either bury it in the calcaneus or bring it back upon itself at a higher level.

Irrigate the surgical wound with Garamycin solution, cauterize identifiable vessels with the electrocautery, and begin closure. Close the peroneal sheath with an absorbable suture and reapproximate the subcutaneous tissues loosely, but again with an absorbable suture. Finally, close the skin with a #4–0 clear nylon subcuticular stitch. Throughout the closure, maintain the foot at a right angle. Apply Steri-strips and place the patient in a well-padded posterior medial plaster splint, which will allow for better control of postoperative edema than will a cast.

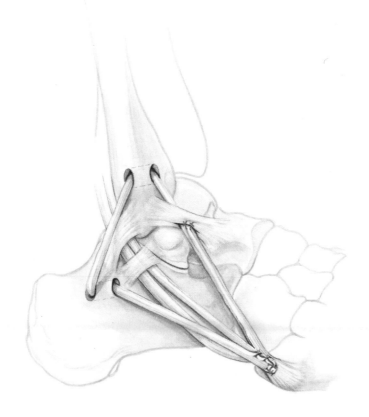

FIGURE 21-10. Sutures are placed at all stress points to secure fixation of the graft.

Postoperative Care and Rehabilitation

Start the patient on nonweightbearing crutch ambulation on the first postoperative day. Have him return to the office in 2 weeks for reevaluation and wound inspection. At that time, place him in a short leg cast, which is maintained for another 6 weeks. After cast removal the patient is placed in an ankle lacer, and rehabilitation is started (Chap. 23).

References

Brostrom Procedure for Reconstruction

1. Brostrom L: Anatomic lesions in recent sprains. *Acta Chir Scand* 1966;132:551.

Chrisman-Snook Procedure for Reconstruction

2. Chrisman OD, Snook GA: Reconstruction of lateral ligament tears of the ankle. *J Bone Jt Surg* 1969;51A:904–912.
3. Elmslie RG: Recurrent subluxation of the ankle joint. *Ann Surg* 1934;100:364–367.

Additional Reading

Balduini FC, Tetzlaff J: Historical perspectives on injuries of the ligaments of the ankle. *Clin Sports Med* 1982;1:3–12.
Brand RL, Collins MD: Operative management of ligamentous injuries to the ankle. *Clin Sports Med* 1982;1:117–130.
Cox JS: Surgical treatment of ankle sprains. *Am J Sports Med* 1977;5:250–251.
Harrington KD: Degenerative arthritis of the ankle secondary to longstanding lateral ligament instability. *J Bone Jt Surg* 1979;61-A:354–361.
Savastano AA, Lowe EB: Ankle sprains: Surgical treatment for recurrent sprains.

Report of 10 patients treated with the Chrisman-Snook modification of the Elmslie procedure. *Am J Sports Med* 1980;8:208–211.

Snook GA, Chrisman OD, Wilson TC: Long term results of the Chrisman-Snook operation for reconstruction of the lateral ligaments of the ankle. *J Bone Jt Surg* 1985;67-A:1–7.

St. Pierre RK, Andrews L, et al: The Cybex II evaluation of lateral ankle ligamentous reconstructions. *Am J Sports Med* 1984;12:52–56.

Vainionpaa S, Kirves P, Laike E: Lateral instability of the ankle and results when treated by the Evans procedure. *Am J Sports Med* 1980;8:437–439.

Treatment of Osteochondritis Dissecans of the Talus

22

Lewis A. Yocum

General Considerations

Osteochondritis dissecans of the talus and osteochondral fracture of the talus are frequently difficult to distinguish one from the other. Trauma is suspected to be a cause, or at least a contributing factor, in the etiology of both. Generally, in the younger individual, a conservative posture is indicated. In addition, the anatomical location of a lesion will influence the decision whether to resort to surgery or not. Berndt and Hardy have classified osteochondritis dissecans of the talus into four stages.[1-4] Assuredly, a Stage IV injury, which involves a displaced fragment, should undergo surgical exploration.[1] Because lateral lesions occur secondary to trauma and rarely heal, they are more likely to call for an aggressive surgical posture in treating them. If a patient opts for conservatism, however, he should be prepared to be immobilized for an extended period of time.

Surgical Procedure and Techniques

In approaching lateral lesions of the talus, place the patient in a supine position on the operating room table. Prep the entire leg and foot and drape them in the usual fashion. Exsanguinate the leg with an Esmarch bandage and hemostatic cuff inflated to 100 mm Hg above systolic pressure (generally, 250 mm Hg).

Using a standard curvilinear anterolateral surgical approach, make the incision just medial to the crest of the fibula and approximately 5 cm from the ankle joint (Fig. 22–1). Carry this incision distally in a curvilinear fashion, coursing over the anterior aspect of the tibiotalar joint and extending it distally

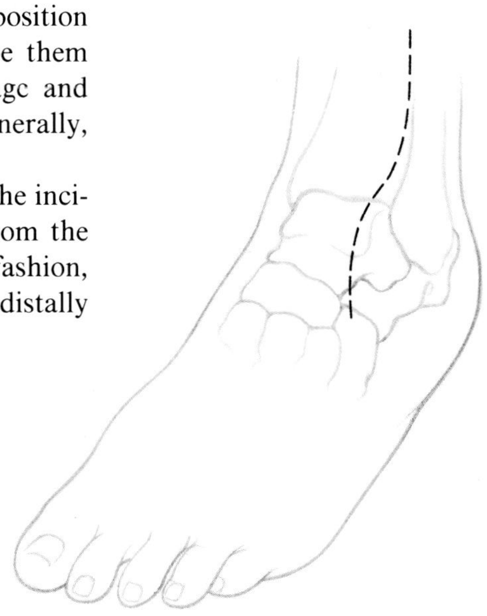

FIGURE 22-1

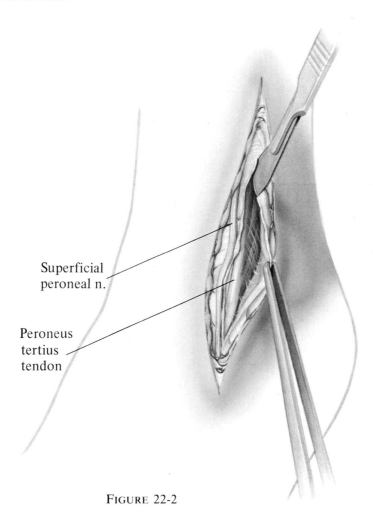

Superficial
peroneal n.

Peroneus
tertius
tendon

FIGURE 22-2

to the level of the sinus tarsi. Carry the dissection down through the subcutaneous tissue and incise the transverse crural and cruciate crural ligaments. Take care throughout the dissection to preserve the cutaneous branches of the superficial peroneal nerve (Fig. 22–2). On entering the ankle joint, also take care to identify the malleolar and lateral tarsal arteries; they are frequently transected in the course of the dissection.

Use blunt dissection to expose as much of the ankle joint as necessary, taking care to preserve the anterior tibiofibular ligament. With dorsiflexion and plantarflexion of the foot, most lesions can be brought into view. Force the foot into inversion to expose the lesion (Fig. 22–3A).

Once identified, approach the osteochondral lesion and outline the extent of the lesion. Naturally, if you encounter a free fragment, this should be removed. Cut the edges of the lesion at a right angle to the talus, curette the base of the lesion, and drill holes with a smooth 0.45 Kirschner wire into the bone at the base of the lesion (Fig. 22–3B,C). "In situ" larger lesions that are still attached should be pinned to the talus. Again, it is advantageous to curette the base and to reattach the larger fragment with pins. Generally, surgical excision and curettement of the base provides more favorable results.

When completed, irrigate the wound with a Garamycin solution. Close the synovium with interrupted absorbable sutures, reestablish the continuity of the crural ligaments, and close the subcutaneous tissues and skin in a routine fashion. In dealing with medial lesions, employ an anteromedial ap-

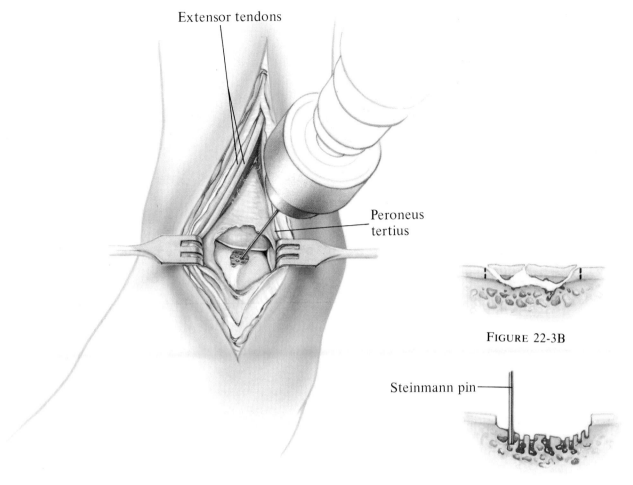

Extensor tendons

Peroneus
tertius

FIGURE 22-3A.   Inversion exposes defect.

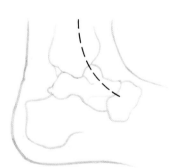

FIGURE 22-3B

Steinmann pin

FIGURE 22-3C

proach and make a curvilinear incision just anterior to the medial malleolus (Fig. 22–4).

Quite often, however, an osteotomy of the medial malleolus is necessary to provide adequate exposure. If this is the case, place a drill hole through the medial malleolus into the tibia (Fig. 22–5). Use a malleolar screw to course through the drill hole and then back it out. Carry an osteotomy obliquely through the medial malleolus at the level of the mortise and expose the tibiotalar joint (Fig. 22–6).

Again, approach the osteochondral lesion and take appropriate care. Following treatment of the lesion, reattach the medial malleolus using the malleolar screw (Fig. 22–7). Close the subcutaneous tissue and skin in the usual fashion. Again, use a compression dressing and place the patient in a posteromedial plaster splint.

FIGURE 22-4

Postoperative Recovery and Rehabilitation

Institute 2 weeks of nonweightbearing crutch ambulation. If an osteotomy has been performed, place the patient in a short leg cast and extend the period of nonweightbearing crutch ambulation. If the patient has not undergone an osteotomy, leave the patient free of a cast so that an early range of motion to the ankle can be initiated, but protect the patient with crutches and do not allow weightbearing for at least 8 weeks. Then start rehabilitation of the lower extremity as outlined in Chapter 23.

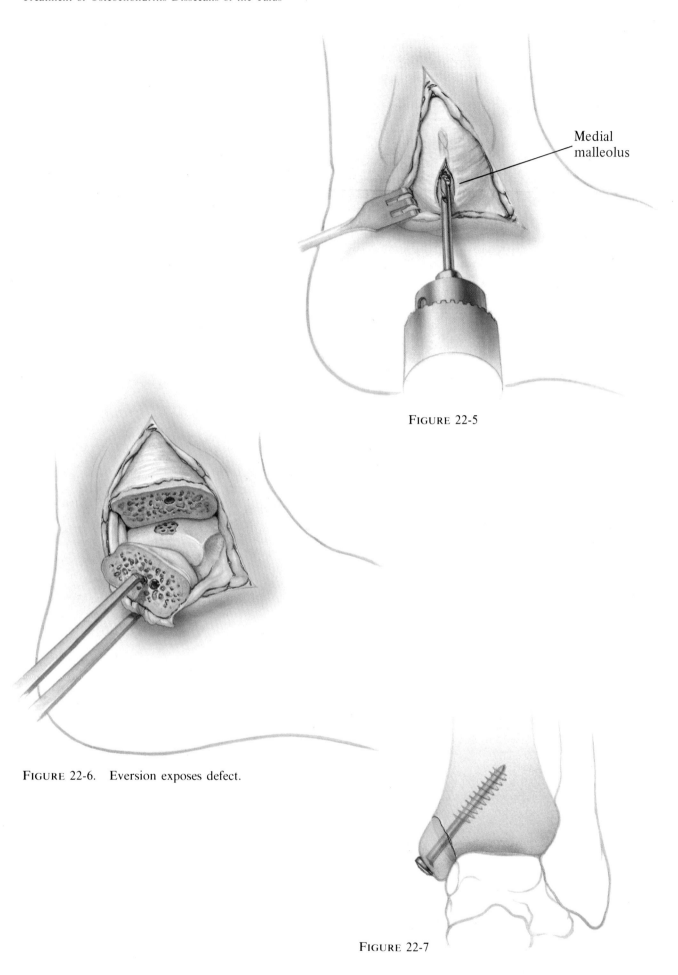

Medial
malleolus

FIGURE 22-5

FIGURE 22-6. Eversion exposes defect.

FIGURE 22-7

References

1. Berndt AL, Harty M: Transchondral fractures (osteochondritis dissecans) of the talus. *J Bone Jt Surg* 1954;41A:988–1020.
2. McCullough CJ, Venugopal V: Osteochondritis dissecans of the talus: The natural history. *Clin Orthop* 1979;144:264–268.
3. Scharling, M: Osteochondritis dissecans of the talus. *Acta Orthop Scand* 1978;49:89–94.
4. Alexander AH, Lichtman DM: Surgical treatment of transchondral Talar-dome fractures (osteochondritis dissecans) *J Bone Jt Surg* 198;62A:646–652.
5. Canale ST, Belding R: Osteochondral lesions of the talus. *J Bone Jt Surg* 1980;62-A:97–102.
6. Mukherjee SK, Young AB: Dome fracture of the talus, a report of ten cases. *J Bone Jt Surg* 1973;55B:319–326.

Additional Reading

O'Farrell TA, Costello BG: Osteochondritis dissecans of the talus. The late results of surgical treatment. *J Bone Jt Surg* 1982;64-A:494–497.

Rynn M. Fazekas EA, Hecker RL: Osteochondral lesions of the talus. *J Foot Surg* 1983;22:155–158.

Thompson JP, Loomer RL: Osteochondral lesions of the talus in a sports medicine clinic, a new radiographic technique and surgical approach. *Am J Sports Med* 1984;12:460–463.

Yuan HA, Cady RB, Derosa C: Osteochondritis dissecans of the talus associated with subchondral cysts. *J Bone Jt Surg* 1979;61-A:1249–1251.

23 Rehabilitation of the Lower Extremity

Clarence L. Shields, Jr., Clive E. Brewster, and Matthew C. Morrissey

Measures to treat or repair the athlete's injured lower extremity are only the necessary first steps in returning him or her to competition. The athlete also needs a full and appropriate course of rehabilitation. Exercises should be performed with constant consideration for the presence or absence of pain. If pain persists, this may indicate an incorrect performance of each exercise. Indeed, in applying any set of specific exercises, it is always best to perform an exercise using sound principles of mechanics against less resistance. Throughout rehabilitation, emphasize to the patient the importance of reporting any pain experienced during an exercise. With this information, the therapist can determine whether or not to continue that exercise at that time.

Immediate Postoperative Rehabilitation

Frequently, the injury is severe and surgical intervention is required. When this is the case, the surgeon should tell the athlete at the outset that the surgical procedure has two phases. Phase I is the actual operation; Phase II, the rehabilitation protocol. Both are equally important. A direct line of communication between surgeon and therapist is essential.

In the initial prescription to the therapist, the surgeon must do these three things: (1) name the surgical procedure; (2) summarize the operative findings; and (3) detail any precautions to be observed during the sequence of exercise routines that are to follow. For example, caution in prescribing progressive resistance exercise is necessary since they may well aggravate any prior condition of lumbar disc herniation in the athlete. Also, throughout the recovery, the therapist keeps a careful and systematic chart of the progress made—including all problems as soon as they are detected—and suggests modifications of the treatment protocol.

If the injured athlete hopes to return to full competition, he or she must undergo a tightly disciplined program of rehabilitation. This is the only way of restoring strength, flexibility, and endurance to all muscles of the lower extremity and of regaining confidence completely. Further, an incompletely rehabilitated extremity, lower or upper has a higher potential for reinjury. Thus, immediate postoperative, and continuing rehabilitation all have three basic goals at every step of the way: (1) to decrease swelling and pain; (2) to restore the full range of motion; and (3) to help the athlete regain adequate strength and self-assurance in that strength.

Immobilized Extremity

Several authors have demonstrated the adverse effect of immobilization at the tissue level. Costill demonstrated a significant decrease in oxidative enzyme systems.[1] Haggmark described the selective atrophy that occurs in Type I slow-twitch muscle fibers during casting.[2] Eriksson showed that electrical stimulation can alter these changes.[3] He concluded that it not only reduces atrophy and weakness but also augments oxidative enzyme activity in the muscle.

When electrical stimulation is going to be used during the immobilization period, it is important first to have the patients go through a trial of electrical stimulation to allay their apprehension and to ensure proper electrode placement.[4] Place one electrode proximally at the femoral triangle and the other in the middle or distal portion of the vastus medialis muscle. Because the distal motor point varies, move the position of the distal electrode until the strongest and most comfortable quadriceps contraction is elicited.

Studies have indicated that static or isometric exercises can produce strength gains.[5,6] These benefits are not as dramatic as those achieved by isotonic exercises, but they are very practical during immobilization. Isometric exercises can be started in the immediate postoperative period. When the patient is comfortable and is still immobilized, add to her program, leg lifts, hip abduction, and hip extension leg exercises.[7]

Nonimmobilized Portions of the Body

If the ankle is not included in the cast, instruct the patient in toe raises. To perform toe raises the patient should stand and lean against a table or a wall for support. They are initiated with body weight alone (e.g., Fig. 23–9). Once these exercises are done with ease, have the patient add equal amounts of weight in each hand. These free-weight exercises can gradually be increased from 10 to 20 pounds with two sets of 25 repetitions.

Vigorous exercising of the contralateral extremity has been shown to produce a "crossover" strengthening effect in the casted limb. Animal studies have demonstrated as much as a 30 percent increase in strength due to this effect.[8-10] Upper body conditioning can be maintained by circuit training on nautilus gym equipment. Single-leg stationary bike riding can also be utilized for cardiac endurance.

Determining Rehabilitative Goals

In order to determine the specific goals for each individual presenting with an injury, a complete evaluation is mandatory. In taking the medical history of the patient, include information regarding any other medical illness for which the patient is currently taking any medication. Include the age and sex of the athlete, the sports in which he or she has participated and wishes to participate in once again, and the level of competition previously attained in each sport. Record not only the date of the most recent injury and the dates of any previous injuries but the date of the athlete's last evaluation by a physician. And be certain to specify the type and length of any prior immobilization of the extremity and its weightbearing status.

In treating patients who have had a surgical procedure, pay very close attention to any chondromalacia found during surgery. Note the presence or absence of the menisci in addition to the amount and location of any degenerative joint disease. And pay special attention to the status of cruciate ligaments and to any other ligamentous laxity found during the surgical procedure.

The next portion of the evaluation is the physical examination. This begins by taking the girth measurements. First, seat the patient, with legs extended, on the table and record the thigh circumference at 20 cm and at 5 cm proximal to the superior border of the patella. Next, measure the calf at the distance of 15 cm distal to the inferior pole of the patella. The most proximal and distal measurements give an indication of the amount of atrophy; the measurement taken at 5 cm, which is closest to the joint, gives an indication of the amount of swelling that is present. Finally, using a goniometer, record the range of motion for flexion and extension, both actively and passively.

An important aspect of the physical evaluation is the patient's pain level. Have the patient rate the level of perceived pain on a scale of zero to 10. Palpate the knee gently to determine the present location of the pain and ask the patient to rate it after each palpation. Next, question the patient about pain that is present with activity, whether it occurs while walking level or on stairs. Finally, record the patient's rating of pain during both quadriceps and hamstring resistance exercises. Another important aspect of the physical evaluation is the presence or absence of sensation near the surgical incisions. Areas of anesthesia can readily be determined by an evaluation of light touch perception.

In evaluating the patient's gait as he or she walks toward you, note the use of any assistive devices such as crutches, canes, the type of brace utilized, and the presence or absence of a flexion or extension stop. As the final component in making the gait analysis, specify the weightbearing status of the limb as indicated by the physician. Begin muscle evaluation by determining the quality and tone of the vastus medialis muscle during a quadriceps contraction.

Basic Rehabilitation Protocol: The Knee

The basic knee program we have worked out at Kerlan-Jobe Orthopedic Clinic remains our key for rehabilitation of all injuries around this joint. The protocol involves three phases, which can be summarized as starting, intermediate, advanced. Patients move into the next phase only when all the goals of the prior phase are achieved. Usually this occurs at 2- to 3-week intervals. The ideal frequency of treatment is daily with supervision, which can be achieved with professional and college-level athletes. The constraints of time and cost, however, allow most patients to have supervision three times a week and to follow an exercise program at home on the off-days.

The Starting Phase

Warmup
A whirlpool for 10 minutes at a temperature of 100 to 105 degrees Fahrenheit or hotpacks for 10 minutes contribute to muscle relaxation and comfort. The patient should always begin the exercise program with warmup contractions of the target muscle or muscles by using isometrics. For isometrics, the contraction time is 10 seconds, and the relaxation time between contractions is 5 seconds.

Two sets of 10 wall slides are performed with the patient supine on the mat (Fig. 23–1). Position the patient close enough to the wall so that the feet remain in contact with the wall throughout the range of knee motions. Using a towel as a slip cloth, the patient gains an active range of flexion by sliding the injured leg down the wall and returning to the starting position by extending the normal extremity. The patient generates range of motion by allowing gravity to assist the leg in sliding down the wall.

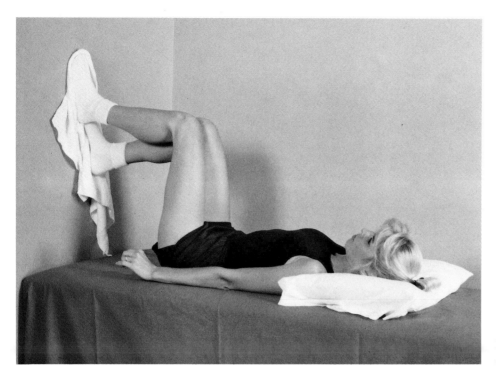

FIGURE 23-1. Wall-slide exercise: Knee.

Hip Exercises

Hip flexion exercises are performed with the patient on the edge of the table with the knee flexed. Have the patient flex the hip without resistance for two sets of 10 repetitions and take a 60-second rest period between sets. Hip abduction is performed with the subject lying on the uninvolved knee with hip flexed (Fig. 23–2). Have the patient extend the involved knee and hip as much as possible, next abduct the injured leg until it is 10 to 14 inches above the mat, then hold this position for a 10-second count, and finally relax the extremity for 5 seconds. Have her perform two series of 10 repetitions. This exercise will contract the gluteus medius muscle as well as the tensor fasciae latae muscle and contribute to lateral knee stability via the iliotibial band. The lateral abdominal musculature is also strengthened when the patient stabilizes the pelvis during hip abduction.[12]

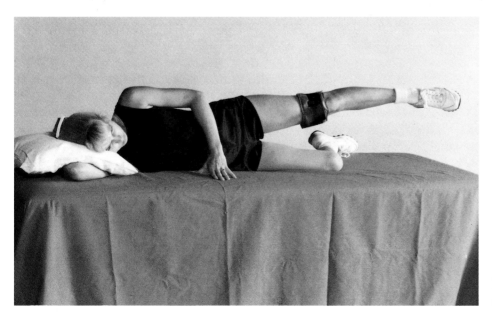

FIGURE 23-2. Abduction exercise: Hip.

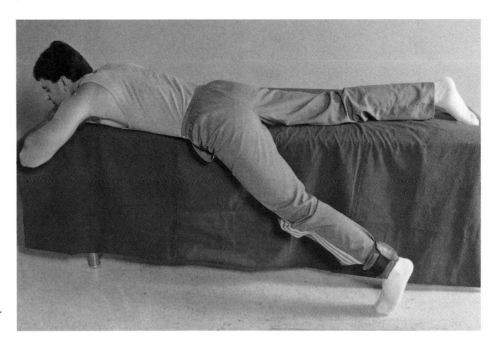

FIGURE 23-3. Extension exercise: Hip.

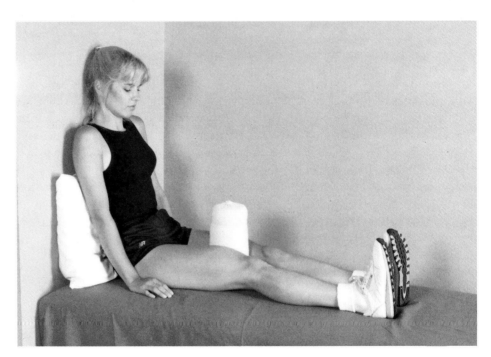

FIGURE 23-4. Adduction exercise: Hip.

Hip extension is done in the prone position with the involved leg over the edge of the mat (Fig. 23–3). Have the patient raise the leg while keeping the knee extended or until the toes of that foot are at mat level. Then, have him hold the position for 10 seconds, relaxing for 2 seconds and continue until two sets of 10 are executed. This motion will exercise the gluteus maximus muscle and also contribute to strengthening of the iliotibial band; in addition, the hamstrings will also be activated as hip extensors. The patient with lower back problems will have difficulty with this exercise, and it may have to be omitted or modified. An alternate method, which concentrates the exercise at the level of the hip, is to flex the knee and relax the hamstrings.

Hip adduction is performed isometrically from the seated position on the mat, the back against a wall (Fig. 23–4). Place a rolled towel between the thighs just above the knee, avoiding any medial knee incisions. Have the

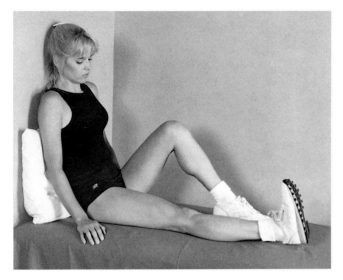

FIGURE 23-5. Quadriceps-setting exercise: Knee.

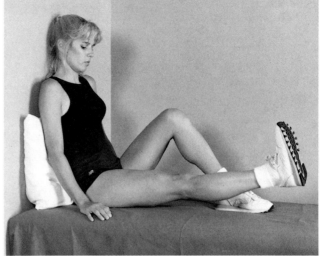

FIGURE 23-6. Straight-leg raise exercise: Knee.

patient adduct the legs with maximal contraction, holding for 10 seconds and relaxing for 5 seconds. Clinically, patients are able to perform quadriceps-setting exercises better if they are started immediately after the hip adduction exercises. This improved performance may occur because the vastus medialis is attached to the adductor tendon.[13] Start the patient on the resistive exercises for the hips with increments of 5 to 10 pounds until he reaches his individual peak. Place weights above the knee to prevent varus force. Adduction and abduction can be performed on Nautilus or Universal Gym equipment after the patient has mastered these particular exercises with the free weights. Hip extension is done with the Nautilus; hip flexion on the Universal.

Knee Exercises

Quadriceps-setting exercises are performed in the seated position and repeated until two sets of 10 have been accomplished (Fig. 23–5). The patient dorsiflexes the foot and toes and pushes the heel away from the body. This seems to help initiate the vastus medialis contraction, which is held maximally for 10 seconds and relaxed for 5 seconds. Electromyographic studies in the Bio-Mechanics Laboratory at Centinela Hospital Medical Center have shown more quadriceps activity during isometric contractions than during simple straight-leg raises. The work of other researchers corroborates this finding.[14,15]

Straight-leg raises are accomplished from the same position (Fig. 23–6). Throughout this exercise, the patient maintains a quadriceps set, which also activates the hip flexors. The patient tightens the quadriceps and holds for 2 seconds, then lifts the entire leg until the heel is 6 inches above the mat. The patient holds the extremity in that position for 2 seconds and then lowers it to the mat for 2 more seconds. This is performed for two sets of 10 repetitions. Add short-arc quadriceps exercises once the patient can tolerate 2 pounds on the straight-leg raises (Fig. 23–7). While the patient is sitting, place a firm pad under the knee to prevent no more than 45 degrees of knee flexion. The patient presses the back of the thigh into the pad as the knee extends and then raises the heel and holds the position for 2 seconds before slowly lowering the leg. The patient completes two sets of 10 repetitions. This produces a concentric contraction, since the muscle is shortening as the knee extends.

Hamstring setting exercises are performed while sitting with 50 to 60 degree of knee flexion (Fig. 23–8). The patient attempts to dig the heel into the

181

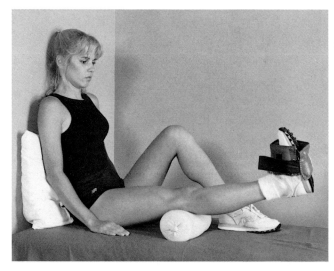

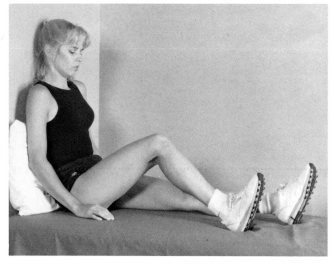

FIGURE 23-7.   Short-arc quadriceps exercise: Knee.

FIGURE 23-8.   Hamstring-setting exercise: Knee.

mat while pulling downward on the leg. Have the patient sustain the hamstring contraction for 10 seconds and then relax for a period of 2 seconds. See that she does two sets of 10 repetitions.

Calf Exercises

Toe raises are initiated with body weight alone, equally distributed on both legs. The patient stands on the floor and braces herself against the wall for support (Fig. 23–9). The plantar flexors of the ankle are held contracted for 10 seconds and then slowly relaxed as the body weight returns to the heel. Twenty-five repetitions are done for each set. As these hip-and-knee exercises

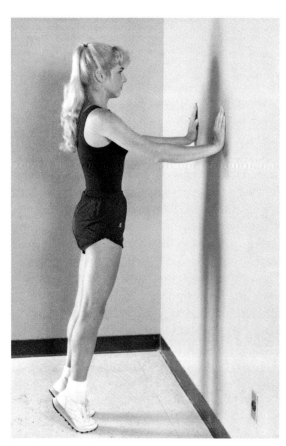

FIGURE 23-9.   Toe-raise exercise: Calf.

182

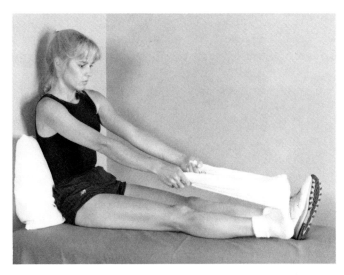

FIGURE 23-10. Towel-stretch: Calf.

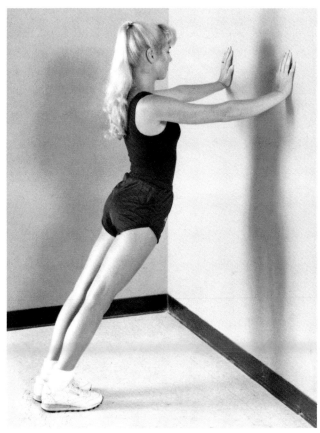

FIGURE 23-11. Gastrocnemius stretch (standing position): Calf.

are repeated, have the weights increased at approximately 2-pound increments until the patient can handle 10 pounds. Next, add resistance to the ankle with a weighted boot. A transfer to Universal Gym equipment or to the Nautilus usually occurs smoothly once this plateau is reached. Add a 5-pound slotted weight to either system, allowing the increases to be in units of 5 rather than 10 pounds. The repetitions are gradually increased up to three sets of 10 repetitions.

Stretching Exercises

Stretching is added when the patient has gained full knee extension. Lengthening of the calf and hamstring muscles are added along with resistance exercises (Fig. 23–10). To do a towel stretch, have the patient sit with back against the wall and the involved leg extended. The patient then loops a towel around the ball of the involved foot and pulls it slowly into dorsiflexion. The calf is stretched if the knee is kept as flat as possible.

Add standing gastrocnemius stretches as the patient can tolerate them (Fig. 23–11). The patient stands approximately 18-inches from the wall with both feet flat on the floor, leans forward while keeping the knees extended, holds the position for 20 seconds and then relaxes 5 seconds. Have both stretches repeated (Figs. 23–10, 23–11) until two sets of 10 repetitions are accomplished. At the end of the workout, ice the knee for 10 minutes to control soreness and swelling.

Free Weights

Ankle weights can be used for isotonic training via straight-leg raises. In the short-arc quadriceps exercises, the range is from a maximum extension to 60 degrees. Add weights in 2-pound increments for both exercises. With each weight load, have the patient perform a set of 10 contractions followed by a 2-minute rest period; have him repeat the set three times. Increase the weights until the strength level of the other leg is reached. This is the maximum weight that the patient can lift and control for 10 repetitions in the same range of motion. The hamstrings can be trained by having the patient lie in the prone position. The leg is worked from the maximum allowable extension to 90 degrees of flexion with the same weight increases. Again, the goal is the maximum weight that can be handled for 10 repetitions in the normal leg. Several authors have outlined isotonic weight protocols.[16,21,23]

Home Program

Performance of the home program is alternated with therapy visits. Have the patient do an active range of motion exercise in the bathtub or pool, perform hip exercises without weights, and work the knee isotonically. Apply ice afterwards. Have her do the same stretches and toe raises and concentrate on normal gait motion. Vigorous pool walking with the water level at the waist will strengthen the upper thigh and lower abdominal muscles.

The Intermediate Phase

Warmup

Once 110 degrees of knee flexion is reached, the patient warms up on the intermediate stage by riding a stationary bicycle with no resistance for 10 minutes. In this phase of rehabilitation, the quadriceps and hamstring musculature are not very well conditioned, and it would be painful to add resistance on the bicycle. It is very important to adjust the seat height so that on the upstroke of the pedal, there are no more then 90 degrees of flexion at the hip and 110 degrees of flexion at the knee.[24] The higher seat level decreases the force on the extensor mechanism. At the downstroke of the pedal, the ankle should have the maximum dorsiflexion that the patient can tolerate. Have the patient continue wall slides (Fig. 23–1) until she has a full range of knee flexion. Have him perform calf stretches from the standing position over a 2 × 9 inch wooden block or a tilt board (Fig. 23–12).

Hip Exercise

Hip adduction and abduction are performed on Nautilus or Universal Gym equipment (Fig. 23–13). Hip extension is done on the Nautilus and hip flexion on the Universal. The resistance is added in 10-pound increments until the strength has reached that of a normal extremity. This is defined as a maximum weight with which a patient can perform two sets of 25 repetitions with a 2-minute rest period between sets.

Knee Exercises

Hamstring curls are done on the Nautilus or Universal (Fig. 23–14). Add eccentric contractions as the patient progresses on the Nautilus. Have the patient lift with both legs and hold the weight with the involved leg for 2 seconds before slowly lowering the weight. This allows the hamstrings to contract while lengthening. Several studies show that more weight can be handled with less effort in an eccentric contraction than in a concentric contraction.[25-27]

Quadriceps resistive exercises are performed in the short arc of zero to 50 degrees, which limits the patellar compressive forces to one-and-a-half

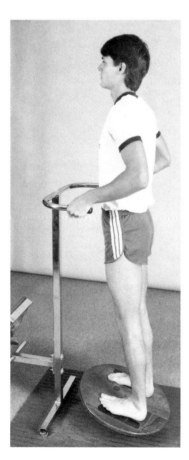

FIGURE 23-12. Tilt-board exercise: Ankle.

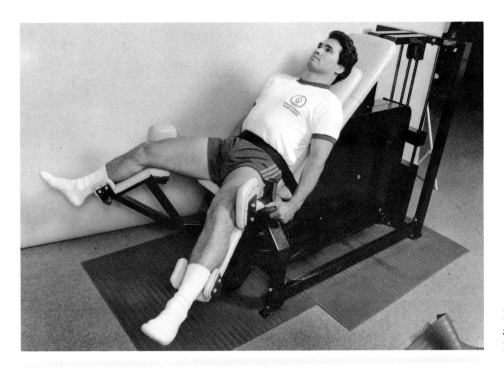

FIGURE 23-13. Adduction and abduction exercise on the Nautilus: Hip.

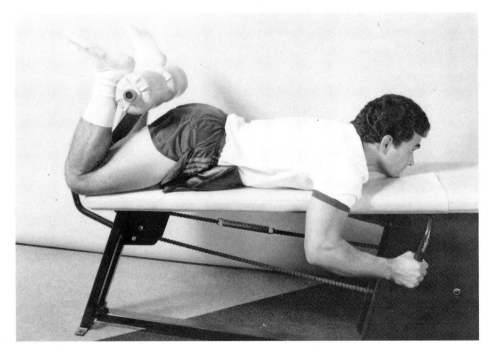

FIGURE 23-14. Hamstring-curl exercise on the Nautilus: Knee.

times the body weight.[28] By having the patient pull the upper pad by hand so that the lower pad rests on the involved leg with the knee as straight as possible (Fig. 23–15), the patient can do eccentric quadriceps contractions on the Universal. The upper pad is then released and the weight held for 2 seconds by the involved leg before being slowly released. These exercises can also be performed on the Nautilus leg-extension machine by raising the weight with both legs and holding for 2 seconds with the involved leg and then lowering with one leg.

Calf Exercise

Step-ups are a form of functional activity that utilizes several muscle groups (Fig. 23–16). The height of the step should not require more than 70 degrees

185

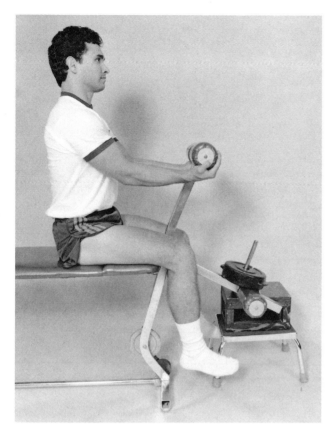

FIGURE 23-15.   Eccentric quadriceps exercise: Knee.

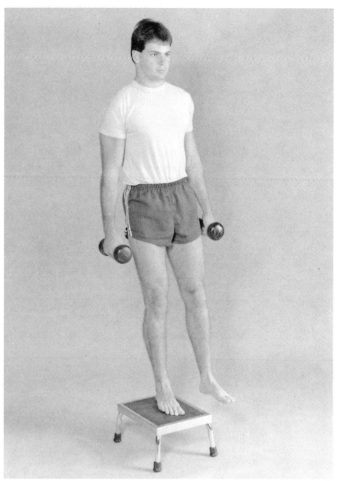

FIGURE 23-16.   Step-up exercise: Knee, Calf.

of knee flexion. This will keep the patellar compressive forces less than two times the body weight. The patient slowly steps up on to the platform with the involved leg first, trying not to push off with the normal leg. In stepping down, the normal leg proceeds first. Start this exercise with just the patient's body weight and then add free weights in 10-pound increments until one-third of the patient's body weight can be handled in two sets of 25 repetitions. The patient should carry dumb bells in either hand as a simple method to perform step-ups. Toe raises are continued with weights on the Universal Gym or Nautilus Machine (Fig. 23–17).

Home Program

The home program continues with the strengthening of the hip, knee, and calf musculature. The patients are instructed to use ankle weights but to keep them at least 10 pounds less than the amount handled in therapy. The patients are warned not to lift weights at home if pain and swelling develop. Toe raises are added along with step-ups. Swimming is beneficial, but if straight-leg kicks are used, have them used cautiously, since patellar pain may develop. Add bicycling to the protocol since both bicycling and swimming are functional exercises. At this point the patient should have enough range of motion for normal gait, but the therapist should observe the gait and correct any deficiencies.

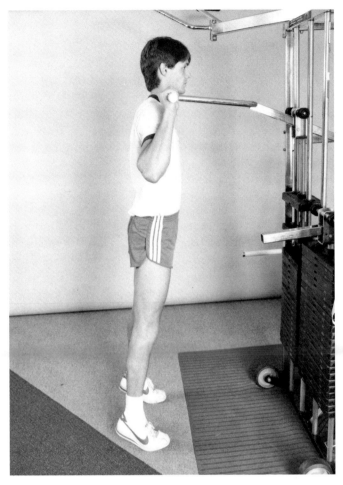

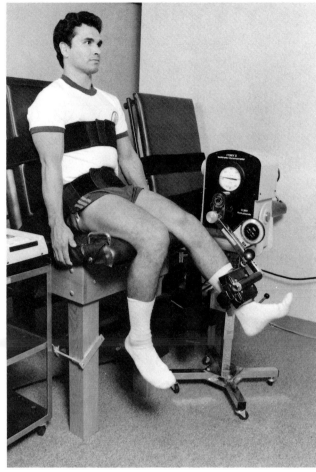

FIGURE 23-17.   Toe-raise exercise on the Universal Gym machine: Calf.

FIGURE 23-18.   Cybex test: Knee.

The Advanced Phase

This phase concentrates on the gradual return to functional activities. Strength and endurance are maximized by using isokinetic machines to train the limb to move at the fast speeds required in athletic competition.

Various Exercises

Wyatt and Edwards suggest that the quadriceps need to be exercised at work rates of 200 and 300 degrees per second to be functionally rehabilitated for just walking.[29] In order to aid the regaining of lateral and rotational mobility, incorporate agility drills at this stage. The patient continues the warmup stretching routines as in the intermediate phase and trains the hip, knee, and calf musculature isotonically until normal strength is achieved. In the hip, and the knee exercises the patient works on the Cybex at a speed of 300 degrees per second for two sets of 20 repetitions (Fig. 23–18). If the Orthotron is used, set it at a speed of 10. In both machines, the speed of the exercises is controlled, either electronically in the former or by hydraulics in the latter. Also, the resistance accommodates to the patient's pain, since no resistance will be met if the limb moves slower than the set speed. Keep the repetitions and sets the same as the isotonic routine, and reduce the speed by increments of 30 degrees per second until 180 degrees per second is reached.

187

Controlled Jogging

To minimize the stresses on the knee start the patient jogging on the trampoline during therapy. This can begin when the injured knee has achieved 80 percent of the quadriceps and hamstring strength of the normal extremity on Cybex testing. This usually corresponds to 1 cm of thigh atrophy at 20 cm above the superior pole of the patella. On the trampoline have the patient start jogging in 5-minute segments, and work until 10 minutes can be tolerated. Then use the treadmill. Beginning with 2-minute sessions, continue until the patient can tolerate 10 minutes of continuous running.

Home Program

In this advanced stage, expand the previous home program to include 5 minutes of running and 5 minutes of walking until the total distance of 1 mile can be covered. Gradually, the running replaces all of the walking, provided there is no swelling or pain. Have the athlete begin agility exercises with figure-of-eight running on a basketball half-court and progressing to "8's" inside the center key. Then start the athlete on backward running, rope skipping, vertical jumps, lateral running and crossovers at a slow pace.[30] When this can be accomplished without pain and swelling, the athlete can now begin practicing the skills of his or her sport. Have the athlete play racquetball (doubles), first, as a way to regain total body coordination. These agility drills should not cause pain and can be performed with increasing speed as the athlete's power and endurance improve.

Cybex Testing

Use Cybex testing to decide when to terminate therapy. Prior training on isokinetic equipment improves an athlete's scores as well as his or her motor-performing skills.[31,32] On the Cybex, an athlete's *strength* is measured as the peak torque he develops at speeds of 180, 240, and 300 degrees per second. An athlete's *power* is measured as the amount of time it takes her to develop a peak torque at each speed. An athlete's *endurance* is the point at which he can no longer produce 50 percent of the original peak torque at a speed of 240 degrees per second.

The athlete can return to his or her sport when strength, power, and endurance are 85 percent of the normal leg. It is very useful to have a preseason Cybex test, since the strength level of both legs may drop after an injury. This visual record of the strength of the involved leg helps the therapist in counseling the athlete.

Competitive Retraining

Once competitors realize that their strength has returned to normal, they can begin a vigorous training program for their respective sports to regain confidence in the injured extremity. Be sure to instruct each rehabilitated competitor in an isotonic program to maintain the strength levels over the next 6 months. The maintenance level is 85 percent of the maximum weight level that the patient achieved at the termination of formal therapy. This requires lifting exercises twice a week in addition to the usual training routine. Bicycle riding or running are good methods of maintaining cardiovascular endurance. And the wearing of a Neoprene rubber sleeve appears to decrease some of the sensitivity that the athlete otherwise experiences when returning to competitive events. Finally, instruct the athlete in a proper warmup and stretching technique.

Rehabilitation Protocols: Special Conditions

Collateral Ligament Sprains

Rehabilitation after injury to the collateral ligament is shorter and progresses with fewer problems than the program for cruciate ligament injury.[33,34] This is due to the decreased severity of the injury as well as the fact that there are no specific strengthening exercises to modify. In the case of medial side lesions, take care during the hip exercises to avoid valgus stress at the knee. Conversely, in the case of lateral ligament injuries, do not allow varus stress to occur. Placing the weights above the knee for the hip exercises will alleviate these loads. The one major problem that occurs during rehabilitation in collateral ligament injuries is the limited range of motion, which is a result of the ligament adhering at the injury site. It may present as a block, either to flexion or to extension, and is more common on the medial side. The therapist must pay close attention to range of motion changes until the full arc of movement is achieved.

Anterior Cruciate Ligament Instability

The anterior cruciate ligament (ACL) functions to prevent both excessive anterior movement of the tibia on the femur and abnormal rotation, internal and external, of the tibia. Larson feels that the ACL functions to guide the knee through its arc of motion.[35] This action allows the other ligaments of the joint to tighten and, in turn, to protect the menisci from excessive force. Several authors have shown that the tension on the ACL is greater from 30 degrees of flexion to full extension.[36] For this reason, we use postoperative casting with knee flexion of 35 to 40 degrees, followed at 6 weeks by bracing with an extension stop of 40 degrees. Intra-articular procedures have to undergo revascularization followed by reorganization of collagen.[37-39] This revascularization and reorganization necessitate a slower and longer process of therapy for these intra-articular procedures, which are followed for 15 weeks before the brace is brought into extension.[40-42] Our studies indicate that a gradual reduction in the flexion contracture, starting at 12 weeks, provides greater stablity for the extra-articular repairs.[43,44]

The primary goal in this rehabilitation is the restoration of dynamic stability by training the muscles that act to prevent excessive tibial rotation in anterior glide on the femur. The muscle group mainly responsible for these functions is the hamstrings. According to Giove, the most valuable finding in ACL rehabilitation is the relationship between the hamstrings quadriceps ratio and the level of sports participation.[45] The basic principle is to strengthen the hamstrings until they are at least of equal strength with the quadriceps on the involved side. This parity allows the athlete to perform at a higher level of activity. The usual ratio quadriceps to hamstrings on the Cybex at a speed of 180 degrees per second is 60:40 (Fig. 23–19).[46] Our goal is to make the hamstring of the involved leg dominant. The optional ratio of 55:45 can be achieved by emphasizing knee flexion throughout therapy (Fig. 23–20).

There are some variations during the starting phase of rehabilitation. For example, perform hip abduction exercises with a hip flexion of 45 degrees when the knee is in 45 degrees of flexion, and place weights above the knee to prevent excess varus load on the knee. For hip extension exercises, one may add weight at the ankle. Increase slightly the flexed posture of the knee beyond that permitted by the brace and thus decrease any tendency of the exercise to result in passive extension. While keeping the quadriceps exercises isometric, advance the hamstrings to resistive exercises. Do not have the patient

189

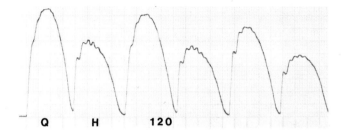

FIGURE 23-19. Normal quadriceps: Hamstring ratio (measurement in foot-pounds of torque).

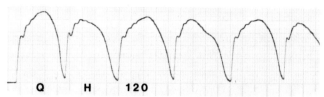

FIGURE 23-20. Hamstring dominant ratio (measurement in foot-pounds of torque).

perform straight-leg raises since they may increase the anterior subluxation of the tibia on the femur. Further studies have demonstrated more electromyographic activity with isometric contractions.[14] Isometric internal and external tibial rotation exercises, which are added once the patient has 90 degrees of knee flexion have been shown to decrease the abnormal tibial rotation that is present.[47] These exercises progress to rubberband resistance.

The intermediate phase features a decrease in the extension stop to 15 degrees. Initiate short-arc quadriceps exercises when the hamstrings are handling 15 pounds. Instruct the patient how to generate a co-contraction of the quadriceps and hamstrings by producing hip extension. Increase both tibial rotations in 5-pound increments on the Universal Gym while the patient is seated in a chair and the knee is flexed to 90 degrees. Give special emphasis to the hamstrings by allowing the patient to do as many as six sets of 10 repetitions. After placing the foot in the loop of the cuff, rotate the tibia internally against the weight (Fig. 23–21).

The advanced phase features eccentric quadriceps exercise and removal of the extension stop. This allows the thigh girth to increase since the quadriceps can produce full knee extension. The rehabilitation for the ACL reconstruction is a very lengthy procedure. An athlete will usually require a year before returning to his or her sport and must also continue to wear a brace for yet another year.

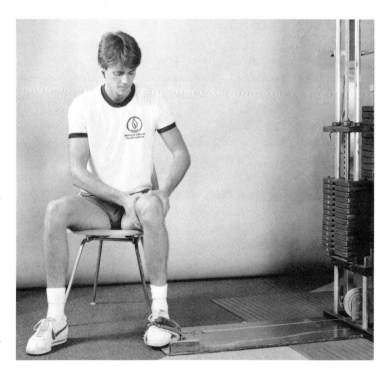

FIGURE 23-21. Internal rotation exercise: Knee.

190

Posterior Cruciate Ligament Instability

The major function of the posterior cruciate ligament (PCL) is to prevent excessive posterior displacement of the tibia on the femur. Hughston considers the ligament to be the primary stabilizer of the knee in flexion, extension, and rotation.[48] He states that in knee motion the tibial plateaus move anteriorly and posteriorly by rotating around the axis of the PCL. A contraction of the quadriceps muscle pulls the tibia anteriorly and thus compensates for the posterior sagging of the tibia. The focus of this rehabilitation is therefore on the quadriceps. Electromyographic studies show that the patients can learn to activate knee extension earlier when running, thus providing stability.[49]

The most common surgical procedure for PCL reconstruction is repositioning of the origin of the medial head of the gastrocnemius muscle.[50] This transfer acts dynamically during the weight acceptance and push-off phases of gait.[51] This can be demonstrated by having the patient maximally contract the gastrocnemius during active plantarflexion of the foot and by watching the tibia move forward from the resting position.

During immobilization, instruct the patient to perform two sets of 20 repetitions of isometric ankle plantarflexion exercises. Do not allow isometric hamstring sets in the cast because they may increase posterior stress on the knee. Have the patient perform straight-leg raises whenever they are tolerated during the cast period.

In the starting phase, advance the quadriceps exercises rapidly while avoiding the hamstring exercises entirely, since they may accentuate the posterior subluxation. Start ankle plantarflexion with two sets of 10 repetitions. Also start eccentric quadriceps exercises as soon as the patient can tolerate them. These exercises, along with step-ups, utilize early the straight-leg raises and short-arc quadriceps exercises. The intermediate phase features resistive quadriceps exercise and avoids stretching the gastrocnemius muscle. Eliminate both the internal and external tibial rotation exercises because they accentuate the posterior subluxation of the tibia. As the patient regains knee extension, start toe raises using body weight; have him do two sets of 20 repetitions. As calf strength improves, add resistance by having the patient hold 10 pounds in each hand. In the advanced phase, the patient progresses to single-leg toe raises. Once the quadriceps have achieved 80 percent of the normal leg on Cybex testing, add hamstring exercises to the program.

Chondromalacia of the Patella

Softening of the patella's articular cartilage may occur from either tracking abnormalities of the patellofemoral joint or spontaneously after a knee injury. Chondromalacia has been attributed to trauma and weakness of the vastus medialis muscle.[28] Contractures of the hamstring muscles are also a common problem in disorders of the patellofemoral joint, and we advise stretching of these muscles to decrease patellar compressive forces. This compression has been documented to rise sharply after 30 degrees of knee flexion and can reach eight times the body weight with a full squat.[52]

Poor muscle contraction can be related during the post-injury period to pain and swelling. Electrical stimulation, when used with ice, is beneficial for its anesthetic and vasoconstricting properties. Simultaneous isometric hip adduction can assist in contractions of the vastus medialis muscle. Since quadriceps-setting and straight-leg raises do not load the patella, continue them throughout the program. Start short-arc quadriceps exercises eccentrically and progress to concentric contractions as tolerated, but limit the range to terminal extensions from zero to 30 degrees. Add hamstring sets and progress to hamstring curls as tolerated, while limiting the flexion to 90 degrees. Hip abductors are not used in patellar-tracking problems since increasing their strength may yield an increase in lateral patellar forces via the linkage to the iliotibial band.

If the patient cannot tolerate the short-arc quadriceps exercise, continue straight-leg raises to 20 pounds.[53] Then have the athlete try the Cybex at speeds of 300 degrees per second. At this high speed, the patella stays in contact with the femoral groove only briefly. Low resistance bicycle exercising is performed with the seat elevated to decrease knee flexion and resultant patellar loading. Add jogging and agility drills as tolerated.

Ankle Injuries

The ankle is the most frequently injured joint in athletics. The lateral collateral ligament reconstructions require a period of nonweightbearing ambulation, which will weaken the musculature of the entire lower extremity. After weightbearing ambulation has started, the hip and thigh musculature can undergo rehabilitation. The initial therapy visits are started with 20 minutes of ice. The cold produces vasoconstriction, which results in decreased edema. in addition, the cold acts as a local anesthetic, which aids in the control of pain and relieves muscle spasm. This is followed by 10 minutes of heat in the form of a hot whirlpool (100°F). A range of active motion exercises are added as the patient can tolerate them. Emphasis should be on dorsiflexion and eversion, while plantarflexion and inversion should be avoided in this early phase to allow healing.

Have the patient perform isometric dorsiflexion by sitting on a mat with outstretched legs and placing the normal foot on the dorsal surface of the injured foot (Fig. 23–22). While applying firm resistance with the top leg, the athlete attempts to dorsiflex the involved ankle. She sustains contraction for 10 seconds, followed by a 5-second relaxation. Have her perform this exercise in two sets of 10 repetitions.

The athlete performs the isometric eversion exercise while sitting in a chair. Have him position the involved leg with 90 degrees of knee flexion and place

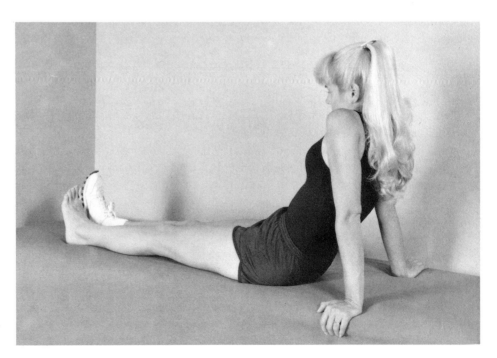

FIGURE 23-22. Isometric dorsiflexion exercise: Ankle.

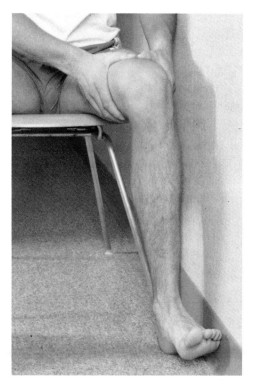

FIGURE 23-23. Isometric eversion exercise: Ankle.

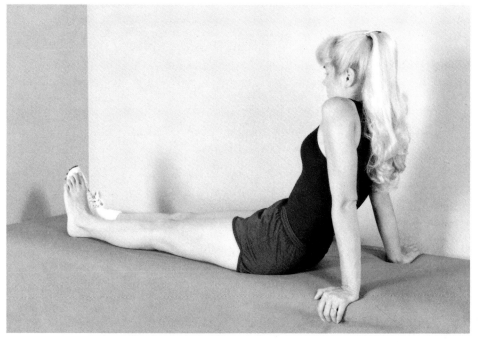

FIGURE 23-24. Isometric plantarflexion exercise: Ankle.

the lateral side of the foot against a wall (Fig. 23–23). Holding the foot flat on the floor, the patient tries to evert the foot against the wall. The movement is held for 10 seconds and relaxed for 5 seconds. The patient accomplishes two sets of 10 repetitions.

As the patient achieves a greater range of pain-free motion, isometric plantar-flexion is added. The patient, sitting on a mat with outstretched legs, places the normal foot under the sole of the injured foot and plantarflexes the involved ankle against the resistance of the normal foot (Fig. 23–24). The patient holds the contraction for 10 seconds, relaxes for 5 seconds, and continues to perform two sets of 10 repetitions. Isometric inversion is added as tolerated by the patient's pain level. The patient, seated in a chair with 90 degrees of knee

193

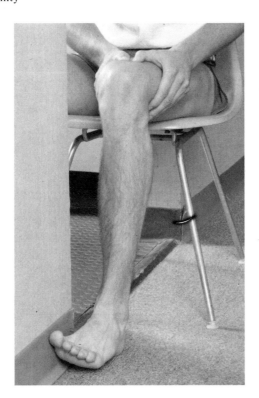

FIGURE 23-25. Isometric inversion exercise: Ankle.

flexion, performs this exercise by placing the medial side of the involved foot against the wall. Holding the foot flat against the floor, the patient inverts the ankle against the wall's resistance (Fig. 23–25). The contraction is maintained for 10 seconds and released for 5 seconds. The patient performs two sets of 10 repetitions.

Once the patient can generate a maximal isometric contraction, add intermediate-phase resistance exercises to the program. At this stage, a thick rubberband is very useful, since the patient can control the resistance he has to work against by varying the amount of stretch in the rubberband. Have the patient perform eversion by sitting in a chair with 90 degrees of knee flexion. Place one end of the rubberband around a stationary object and loop the free end around the lateral side of the foot at the metatarsal head area (Fig. 23–26). While the heel remains in contact with the floor, the patient everts the foot against the rubberband. The contraction is held for 2 seconds; then the foot is returned to the starting position. The resistance can be increased by applying more stretch to the rubberband. Have the patient perform two sets of 10 repetitions. Inversion exercises are executed from the same position. The only difference is that the free end of the rubberband is around the medial side of the foot. The sets and repetitions are the same.

The patient performs plantarflexion resistive exercises while sitting on a mat with outstretched legs. Loop the end of the rubberband around the sole of the foot while the patient holds the other end in the palm of the hand on the same side of the body (Fig. 23–27). For example, the right foot is teamed with the right hand. The patient performs two sets of 10 repetitions.

During dorsiflexion resistive exercises, the patient sits on a mat with the legs extended. Place one end of the rubberband around a stable object (e.g., a table edge) and loop the free end around the dorsum of the foot. The foot is dorsiflexed against the resistance of the rubberband (Fig. 23–28). Two sets of 10 repetitions are performed by the athlete. Add toe raises (Fig. 23–9) and heel-cord stretching (Fig. 23–11) as the patient can tolerate them. Finally,

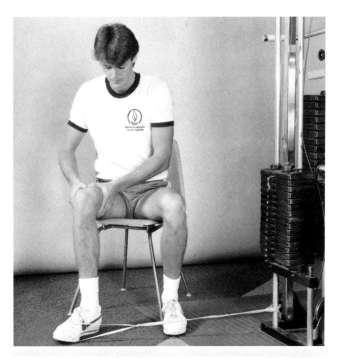

FIGURE 23-26. Everson exercise: Ankle.

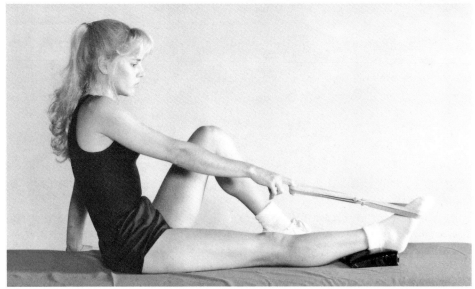

FIGURE 23-27. Plantarflexion exercise: Ankle.

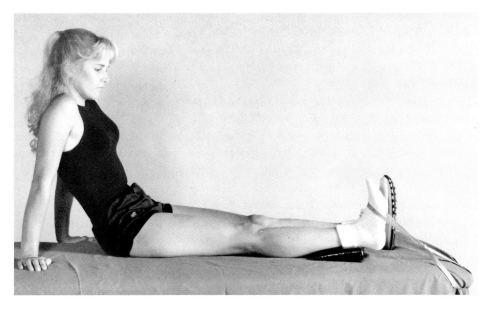

FIGURE 23-28. Dorsiflexion exercise: Ankle.

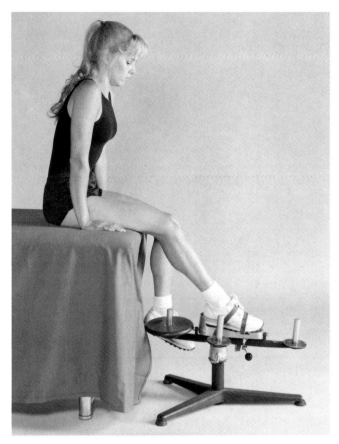

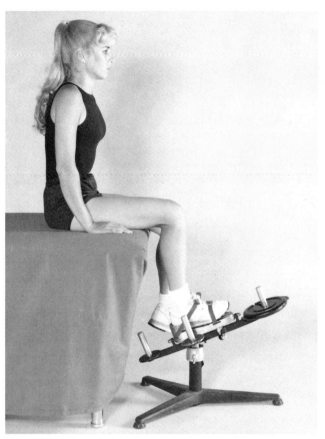

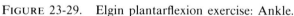

FIGURE 23-29.   Elgin plantarflexion exercise: Ankle.

FIGURE 23-30.   Elgin dorsiflexion exercise: Ankle.

add the rockerboard to increase the range of ankle motion and to assist in recovering proprioception (Fig. 23–12).

In the advanced phase, the patient will work against weights using the Elgin ankle machine. Emphasize ankle eversion exercises by allowing the patient to perform three sets of 10 repetitions. Add weights in 2-pound increments and increase the load until normal ankle strength is achieved. Seat the athlete with the hip and knee flexed 90 degrees and the foot strapped securely into the exerciser in the neutral position. For plantarflexion exercises, place the weight posteriorly to the heel (Fig. 23–29) and have the patient plantarflex the ankle against the resistance of the weight. After completion of this exercise, transfer the weight anteriorly to the toes and have the patient dorsiflex the ankle weights (Fig. 23–30).

The patient performs eversion exercises with the weight on the lateral side of the foot (Fig. 23–31); she performs inversion resistance exercises with the weight on the medial side of the foot (Fig. 23–32). If the ankle exercise machine is not available, Velcro strap weights can be used as an alternative. To perform ankle inversion exercises, the patient lies on his injured side on the exercise table (Fig. 23–33). Strap a 2-pound weight around the foot at arch level. The patient then raises the foot toward the ceiling without moving the lower leg. Have the patient perform ankle eversion exercises by lying on the normal side and everting the foot (Fig. 23–34). To perform ankle dorsiflexion, the patient sits on the end of the table, though his foot must not touch the floor (Fig. 23–35). The patient dorsiflexes the weight for two sets of 10 repetitions. Ankle plantarflexion progresses by single-leg toe raises. The Cybex can also

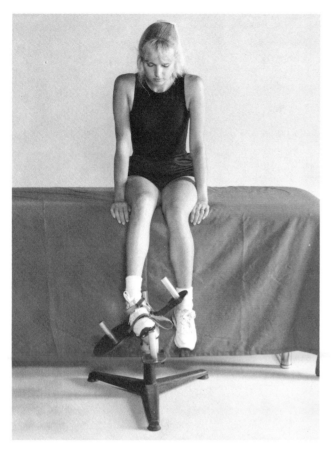

FIGURE 23-31.   Elgin eversion exercise: Ankle.

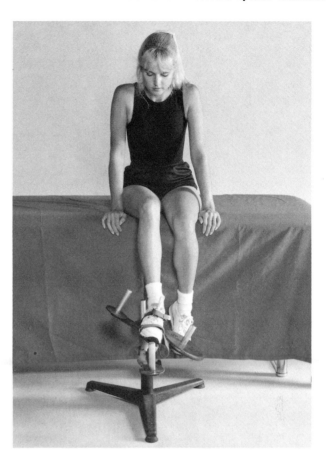

FIGURE 23-32.   Elgin inversion exercise: Ankle.

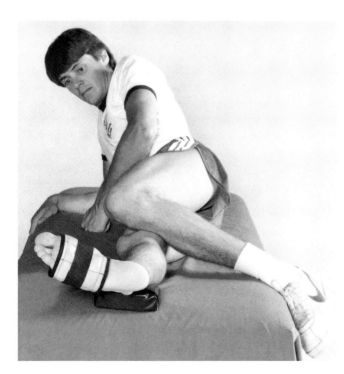

FIGURE 23-33.   Inversion exercise: Ankle.

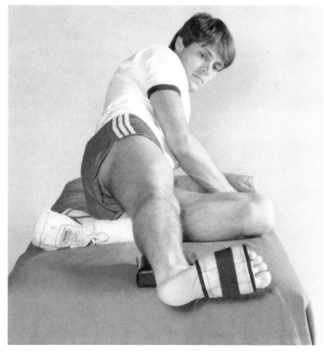

FIGURE 23-34.   Eversion exercise: Ankle.

be utilized for all the ankle resistance exercises. Start the patient on the basic jogging program and have him progress to agility drills as tolerated. For these activities, the ankle must always be taped.

197

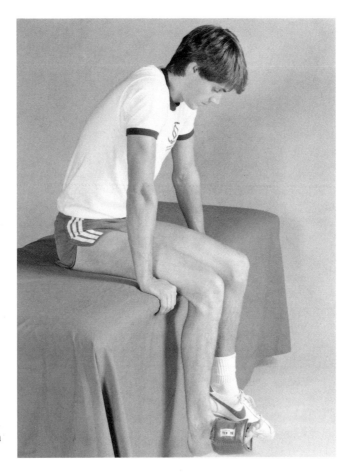

FIGURE 23-35. Dorsiflexion exercise: Ankle.

References

1. Costill DL, Fink WJ, et al: Muscle rehabilitation after knee surgery. *Phys Sports Med* 1977;5(9):71–74.
2. Haggmark TN, Eriksson E: Cylinder or mobile cast brace after knee ligament surgery. A clinical analysis and morhologic and enzymatic studies of changes in the quadriceps muscle. *Am J Sports Med* 1979;7:48–56.
3. Eriksson E, Haggmark T; Comparison of isometric muscle training and electrical stimulation supplementing isometric muscle training in the recovery after major knee ligament surgery. *Am J Sports Med* 1979;7:169–171.
4. Gould N, Donnermeyer D, et al: Transcutaneous muscle stimulation as a method to retard disuse atrophy. *Clin Orthop* 1982;164:215–220.
5. Grimby G, Gustafsson E: Quadriceps function and training after knee ligament surgery. *Med Sci Sports Exerc* 1980;12:70–75.
6. Rasch PJ, Morehouse LE: Effect of static and dynamic exercises on muscular strength and hypertrophy. *J Appl Physiol* 1957;11:29–34.
7. Steadman JR: Rehabilitation of athletic injuries. *Am J Sports Med* 1979;7:147–149.
8. Hellebrandt FA, Houtz SJ, et al: Influence of bimanual exercise on unilateral work capacity. *J Appl Physiol* 1950;2:446–452.
9. Hellebrandt FA, Waterland JC: Indirect learning. The influence of unimanual exercise on related muscle groups of the same and the opposite side. *Am J Phys Med* 1962;41:45–55.
10. Hellebrandt FA, Houtz SJ, et al: Tonic neck reflexes in exercises of stress in man. *Am J Phys Med* 1956;35:144–159.
11. Nicholas J, Scott N, et al: Rehabilitation of the knee. In Helfet AJ (ed), *Disorders of the Knee*, ed 2. Philadelphia, Lippincott, 1982, pp 469–475.
12. Bose K, Kanagasuntheram R, et al: Vastus medialis oblique: An anatomic & physiologic study. *Orthopedics* 1980;3:880–883.

13. Rosentswieg J, Hinson MM: Comparison of isometric isotomic and isokinetic exercises by electromyography. *Arch Phys Med Rehabil* 1972;53:249–252.
14. Lieb FJ, Perry J: Quadriceps function: An electromyographic study under isometric contraction. *J Bone Jt Surg* 1971;53-A:759–758.
15. Smith MJ, Melton P: Isokinetic vs isotonic variable resistance training. *Am J Sports Med* 1981;9:275–279.
16. Lesmes GR, Costill DL, et al: Muscle strength and power changes during maximal isokinetic training. *Med Sci Sports Exerc* 1978;10:266–269.
17. Sherman WM, Pearson DR, et al: Isokinetic rehabilitation after surgery. A review of factors which are important for developing physiotherapeutic techniques after knee surgery. *Am J Sports Med* 1982;10:155–161.
18. Perrine JJ, Edgerton VR: Muscle force-velocity relationships under isokinetic loading. *Med Sci Sports* 1978;10:159–166.
19. Coyle EF, Feiring DC, et al: Specificity of power improvements through slow and fast isokinetic training. *J Appl Physiol* 1981;51:1437–1442.
20. Costill DL, Coyle EF, et al: Adaptions in skeletal muscle following strength training. *J Appl Physiol* 1979;46:96–99.
21. Grimby G, Gustafsson E, et al: Quadriceps function and training after knee ligament surgery. *Med Sci Sports Exerc* 1980;12:70–75.
22. Leach RE, Stryker WS, et al: Comparative study of isometric and isotonic quadriceps exercise programs. *J Bone Jt Surg* 1965;47-A:1421–1426.
23. McLeod WD, Blackburn TA: Biomechanics of knee rehabilitation with cycling. *Am J Sports Med* 1980;8:175–180.
24. Standish WD: Treatment of chronic tendinitis with eccentric exercise training. Presented at the annual meeting of the American Academy of Orthopaedic Surgeons, Las Vegas, NV Feb 24, 1981.
25. Johnson BL: Eccentric vs concentric muscle training for strength development. *Med Sci Sports* 1972;4:111–115.
26. Mannheimer JF: A comparison of strength gain between concentric and eccentric contractions. *Phys Ther* 1969;49:1201–1207.
27. Outerbridge RE, Dunlop JA: The problem of chondromalacia patallae. *Clin Orthop* 1975;110:177–196.
28. Wyatt MP, Edwards AM: Comparison of quadriceps and hamstring torque values during isokinetic exercise. *J Orthop Sports Phys Ther* 1981;3:48–56.
29. Yamamoto SK, Hartman CW: Functional rehabilitation of the knee: A preliminary study. *J Sports Med* 1975;3:288–291.
30. Pipes TV, Wilmore JH: Isokinetic vs isotonic strength training in adult men. *Med Sci Sports* 1975;7:262–274.
31. Pipes TV: Acquisition of muscular strength through constant and variable resistance strength training. *Ath Train* 1977;12:146–148,150–151.
32. Bergfeld J: Functional rehabilitation of isolated medial collateral ligament sprains. *Am J Sports Med* 1979;7:207–209.
33. Steadman JR: Rehabilitation of first and second degree sprains of the medial collateral ligament. *Am J Sports Med* 1979;7:300–302.
34. Larson RL: Editorial, The knee physiological joint. *J Bone Jt Surg* 1983;65-A:143–144.
35. Henning CE, Lynch MA: An in vivo strain gauge study of elongation of the anterior cruciate ligament. *Am J Sports Med* 1985;13:22–26.
36. Clancy WG, Jr., Nelson DA, et al: Anterior cruciate ligament reconstruction using one-third of the patellar ligament, augmented by extra-articulr tendon transfer. *J Bone Jt Surg* 1982;64-A:352–359.
37. Caubad HE, Rodkey WG, et al: Experimental studies of acute anterior cruciate ligament injury and repair. *Am J Sports Med* 1979;7:18–22.
38. Noyes FR, Matthews DS, et al: The symptomatic anterior cruciate deficient knee. Part I, *J Bone Jr Surg* 1983;65-A:154–162.
39. Noyes FR, Matthews DS, et al: The symptomatic anterior cruciate deficient knee. Part II, *J Bone Jt Surg* 1983;65-A:163–174.
40. Cabaud HE, Feagin JA, et al: Acute anterior cruciate ligament injury and augmented repair. Experimental studies. *Am J Sports Med* 1980;8:395–401.

199

41. Paulos L, Noyes FR, et al: Knee rehabilitation after anterior cruciate ligament reconstruction and repair. *Am J Sports Med* 1981;9:140–149.
42. Tacconelli VA, Tibone JE, et al: Intra-articular substitution for anterior cruciate deficient knees: A clinical comparison of three methods. Presented at the winter meeting of the American Orthopaedic Society for Sports Medicine. New Orleans, LA, Jan 1982.
43. Beyer AH, Shields CL: Extra-articular reconstruction of anterior cruciate ligament. Presented at the annual meeting of American Orthopaedic Society for Sports Medicine. Williamsburg, VA, July 1983.
44. Giove TA, Miller SJ: Non-operative treatment of the torn anterior cruciate ligament. *J Bone Jr Surg* 1983;65-A:184–192.
45. Stafford MG, Grana WA: Hamstring/quadriceps ratios in college football players: A high velocity evaluation. *Am J Sports Med* 1984;12:209–211.
46. Slocum DB, Larson RL: Rotatory instability of the knee. Its pathogenesis and a clinical test to demonstrate its presence. *J Bone Jt Surg* 1968;50-A:211–225.
47. Hughston JC, Andrews JR, et al: Classification of the knee ligament instabilities. Part I. The medial compartment and cruciate ligaments. *J Bone Jt Surg* 1976;58-A:159–172.
48. Cain TW, Schwab G: Performance of athletes with straight posterior instability of the knee. Presented at annual meeting of the American Orthopaedic Society for Sports Medicine: Big Sky, MT, June 1980.
49. Kennedy JC, Galpin RD: The use of the medial head of the gastrocnemius muscle in the posterior cruciate-deficient knee. indications—technique—results. *Am J Sports Med* 1982;10:63–74.
50. Insall JN, Wood RW: Bone block transfer of the medial head of the gastrocnemius for posterior cruciate insufficiency. *J Bone Jt Surg* 1982;64-A:691–699.
51. Hungerford DS, Lennox DW: Rehabilitation of the knee in disorders of patellofemoral joint: Relevant biomechanics. *Ortho Clin North Am* 1983;14:397–402.
52. Dehaven KE, Dolan WA, et al: Chondromalacia patella in athletes. *Am J Sports Med* 1979;7:5–11.

Additional Reading

Curl WW, Markey KL, Mitchell WA: Agility training following anterior cruciate ligament reconstruction. *Clin Orthop* 1983;172:133–136.

Montgomery JB, Steadman JR: Rehabilitation of the injured knee. *Clin Sport Med* 1985;4:333–343.

Steadman JR: Rehabilitation of acute injuries of the anterior cruciate ligament. *Clin Orthop* 1983;172:129–132.

Index

Achilles tendon
   complete rupture of, 158–161
      general considerations, 158
      mechanism of injury for, 158
      partial vs, 156
      physical conditioning effects on,
         158
      postoperative care and rehabilitation
         for, 160–161
      site of disruption in, 158
      surgical repair of, 158–160, 159f,
         160f
      Thompson test of, 158
   inflammation of, 155–158
      acute vs chronic, 155
      diagnosis of, 155
      fascial graft reconstruction for, 155,
         156, 157f
      general considerations, 155
      medical treatment of, 155
      nonsteroidal anti-inflammatory drugs
         for, 155
      partial tendon rupture vs, 156
      from prominent os calcis beak, 155,
         157, 158, 158f
      surgical treatment of, 155, 156–
         157, 156–158f
      tendon sheath resection for, 155,
         156, 156f
   partial rupture of, 155–158
      complete vs, 156
      diagnosis of, 156
      fascial graft reconstruction for, 155,
         156, 157f
      general considerations, 156
      postoperative care and rehabilitation
         for, 158
      from prominent os calcis beak, 157,
         158f, 158f
      surgical treatment of, 156–157,
         156–158f
      tendinitis vs, 156

Ankle injuries
   of Achilles tendon. *See* Achilles tendon
   arthroscopy of
      anatomical considerations in, 152
      anesthesia for, 152
      anteromedial and anterolateral ap-
         proach, 152, 153f
      general considerations, 152
      patient position for, 152
      posterolateral approach to, 152,
         153f
      techniques of, 152–153, 153f
   exercises for. *See* Exercises for ankle
   of lateral ligament. *See* Lateral liga-
      ment injuries of ankle
   from os calcis beak, 155
   rehabilitative programs for. *See* Reha-
      bilitation programs for ankle
      injuries
   of talus. *See* Talus injuries
Anterior cruciate ligament injuries of
      knee
   acute
      with lateral collateral ligament in-
         jury, 124
      with medial collateral ligament in-
         jury, 111, 114–115, 115f
   chronic
      diagnosis of, 134
      general considerations, 134–135
      with medial collateral ligament in-
         jury, 119, 120
      treatment of, 120, 134–148
   function considerations, 134, 189
   rehabilitation programs for
      immediate postoperative care, 118,
         147–148
      protocols for, 189–190, 190f
   surgical repair of
      iliotibial band transfer in, 135, 138–
         142, 138–141f
      indications for, 134

      with lateral collateral ligament re-
         pair, 124
      with medial collateral ligament re-
         pair, 114–115, 115f
      meniscectomy in, 135
      patellar tendon transfer in, 135,
         142–147, 142–147f
      pes anserinus transfer in, 135–138,
         135–137f
      postoperative care and rehabilitation,
         118, 147–148
      with semilunar cartilage damage,
         135
Arthroscopy
   of ankle injuries
      anatomical considerations in, 152
      anesthesia for, 152
      anteromedial and anterolateral ap-
         proach, 152, 153f
      general considerations, 152
      patient position for, 152
      posterolateral approach, 152, 153f
      techniques of, 152–153, 153f
   of elbow injuries, 40–42
      anterior approach, 41, 41f, 42f
      arm position for, 40–41
      general considerations, 40
      needle injection for, 41
      posterior approach, 40f, 41
      techniques of, 40–42, 40–42f
   of knee injuries, 92–98
      anesthesia for, 92, 93
      arthroscope insertion for, 93, 94f
      cruciate ligament inspection in, 96,
         96f, 97f
      general considerations, 92
      incisions for, 93
      lateral meniscus in, 96
      leg holders for, 93
      ligamentous examination prior to,
         92
      medial meniscus in, 93, 95f

Arthroscopy (cont.)
  patellofemoral joint inspection in,
    93, 94f
  patient position for, 92
  popliteal tendon in, 96, 96f
  portals for, 93, 95, 97
  suprapatellar pouch in, 93
  techniques of, 92–98, 94–97f
  of shoulder injuries, 2–7
    abduction of arm for, 2, 3f
    anatomical considerations for, 2, 4f
    anesthesia for, 3, 4
    anterior approach, 5–7, 6f
    arthroscope insertion, 3–5
    forward flexion of arm for, 2, 3f
    general considerations, 2
    indications for, 2
    needle injection, 3, 4f
    posterior approach, 4, 5f
    pulley system for, 2
    surgical procedures performed via, 7
    techniques for, 2–7, 3–6f
    traction setup for, 2
Axillary nerve, 2, 4f

Bankart lesions
  arthroscopy of, 2
  excision of
    modified Bristow procedure for, 23
    staple capsulorrhaphy for, 27, 34
Biceps tendon
  arthroscopy of, 2, 4, 5f, 6f
  in impingement syndrome, 11, 16–17
  rupture of, surgical repair of
    dissection procedures, 58, 58f
    drilling of holes in bicipital tuberos-
      ity for, 58–59, 59f
    general considerations, 57
    incision technique for, 57, 57f, 58,
      58f
    postoperative care and rehabilitation,
      61
    sutures for, 59, 60f
    techniques of, 57–61, 57–60f
  tenodesis of, 16–18, 17f, 18f
    indications for, 16–17
    techniques of, 17–18, 17f, 18f
Bristow procedure, modified, 20–27
  for Bankart lesion treatment, 23
  arthrotomy in, 23, 24f
  for avulsion fracture, 24
  axillary approach, 20–21
  bone block in, affixment of, 20, 24–
    26, 25f, 27f
  deltopectoral approach, 20–21, 21f
  dissection procedures, 21–24, 22–24f
  drilling of holes in glenoid and cora-
    coid process in, 24–26, 25f
  general considerations, 20
  musculocutaneous nerve considerations
    in, 23, 23f
  patient position for, 20

postoperative care and rehabilitation
  for, 27, 83
screw placement in, 26, 27f
subscapularis muscle splitting in, 23
techniques of, 20–26, 21–25f, 27f
Brostrom procedure for lateral ligament
  reconstruction of ankle
  with avulsion injury, 162, 163
  dissection procedures, 162–163, 163f
  general considerations, 162
  incisions for, 162, 163f
  objectives of, 162
  postoperative care and rehabilitation,
    165
  techniques of, 162–165, 163–165f

Calcaneofibular ligament reconstruction
  Brostrom procedure, 162, 164f
  Chrismon-Snook procedure, 165
Chondromalacia of patella, 191–192
Chrisman-Snook procedure for lateral ligament reconstruction of ankle
  anesthesia and leg position for, 166
  general considerations, 165
  incisions for, 166, 166f
  indications for, 165
  peroneus brevis tendon graft in, 166–
    168, 167f, 168f
  postoperative care and rehabilitation
    for, 169
  techniques of, 166–168, 166–169f
Collateral ligaments of elbow
  medial. See Medial collateral ligament
    injuries of elbow
  ulnar, 49
Collateral ligaments of knee
  lateral. See Lateral collateral ligament
    injuries of knee
  medial. See Medial collateral ligament
    injuries of knee
Coracoacromial ligament resection, 8–11
  general considerations, 8–9
  for impingement syndrome, 8–9
  patient position for, 9
  postoperative care and rehabilitation
    for, 10–11
  techniques of, 9–10, 9f, 10f
Cruciate ligaments of knee
  anterior. See Anterior cruciate ligament
    injuries of knee
  dissection of, 112, 113f
  posterior. See Posterior cruciate liga-
    ment injuries of knee

Drawer test, posterior, 111–112

Elbow injuries
  arthroscopy of, 40–42
    anterior approach, 41, 41f, 42f
    arm position for, 40–41

general considerations, 40
needle injection for, 41
posterior approach, 40f, 41
techniques of, 40–42, 40–42f
debridement of loose bodies from, 46–
  48
  general considerations, 46
  incision for, 46, 47f
  indications for, 46
  osteotomy with, 46–48, 47f
  postoperative care and rehabilitation
    for, 48
  techniques of, 46–48, 47f
exercises for. See Exercises for elbow
lateral epicondyle in. See Lateral epicondyle of elbow
of medial collateral ligament. See Medial collateral ligament injuries of
  elbow
medial epicondyle in
  arthroscopy of, 41
  ulnar nerve transfer and, 54
rehabilitation programs for. See Rehabilitation programs for elbow
  injuries
of ulnar collateral ligament, 49
Elgin ankle machine exercises, 196,
  196f, 197f
Ellison procedure for iliotibial band transfer. See Iliotibial band transfer,
  Ellison procedure
Exercises
  for ankle
    after Achilles tendon repair, 160–
      161
    after Brostrom procedure for liga-
      ment reconstruction, 165
    with Cybex machine, 196–197
    dorsiflexion, 192, 192f, 194, 195f,
      196, 196f, 198f
    with Elgin ankle machine, 196,
      196f, 197f
    eversion, 193, 193f, 194, 195f,
      196, 197f
    during immobilization period, 177
    isometric, 192–194, 192–194f
    plantarflexion, 193, 193f, 194,
      195f, 196, 196f
    with Velcro strap weights, 196,
      197f, 198f
  for elbow
    after biceps tendon rupture repair,
      61
    after debridement of loose bodies,
      48
    extension stretch, 78, 78f, 87–88,
      87f, 88f
    finger flexion, 85–86
    flexion stretch, 78, 78f, 85–86, 87,
      87f, 88, 88f
    forearm pronation and supination,
      86, 86f, 88
    radial deviation, 86, 86f

after release of lateral epicondyle, 45
strengthening, 85–87
ulnar deviation, 86
after ulnar nerve transfer, 55
wrist stretches, 85, 85f, 87, 87f
for knee
    after anterior cruciate ligament repair, 147–148, 189–190, 190f
    calf, 182–183, 182f, 185–186, 186f, 187f
    controlled jogging, 188
    with Cybex machine, 187, 187f, 188
    with free weights, 183–184
    gastrocnemius stretching, 183, 183f
    hamstring curls, 184, 185f
    hamstring-setting, 181–182, 182f
    hip abduction, 179, 179f, 181, 184, 185f
    hip adduction, 180, 180f, 181, 184, 185f
    hip extension, 180, 180f, 181, 184
    hip flexion, 179, 181, 184
    home programs, 184, 186, 188
    after iliotibial band transfer, 147–148
    during immobilization period, 177
    after lateral collateral ligament repair, 125, 127
    after medial collateral ligament repair, 120–121
    after patellar realignment, 104
    after patellar tendinitis repair, 106
    after patellar tendon rupture repair, 109
    after patellar tendon transfer, 147–148
    after pes anserinus transfer, 147–148
    after posterior cruciate ligament repair, 133
    quadriceps resistive, 184–185, 186f
    quadriceps-setting, 181, 181f
    short-arc quadriceps, 181, 182f
    step-up, 185–186, 186f
    straight-leg raising, 181, 181f
    stretching, 183, 183f
    tilt-board, 184, 184f
    toe-raising, 182, 182f, 186, 187f
    towel-stretching, 183, 183f
    wall-slide, 178, 179f, 184
    warmup, 178, 179f, 184, 187
for shoulder
    abduction, 73–75, 73f, 74f, 79, 79f, 80f
    adduction, 77, 77f
    anterior capsule stretches, 70–71, 71f
    after anterior reconstruction, 83–84
    after anterior staple capsulorrhaphy, 30, 83
    after coracoacromial ligament resection, 10–11

elbow flexion and extension, 78, 78f
extension, 77–78, 78f
flexion, 73, 73f
home programs, 69, 79
for impingement syndrome, 82–83
inferior capsule stretches, 71, 72f
isometric, 69, 69f
joint mobilization with, 68, 68f
after modified Bristow procedure, 27, 83
pendulum, 64–66, 65f
posterior capsule stretches, 72, 72f
after posterior reconstruction, 84
after posterior staple capsulorrhaphy, 36, 84
progressive resistance, 72–73
rotation stretches, 63–64, 65f
    external, 75–76, 75f
    internal, 76, 76f
after rotator cuff repair, 16, 83
saw, 64, 65f
shrug, 66, 66f, 77
stretches, 63–64, 65f, 70–72, 70–72f
throwing, 81–82
wall slide, 66–67, 66f, 67f
wand, 67, 67f, 68f
warmup, 62–63

Fibulocalcaneal ligament reconstruction
Brostrom procedure, 162, 164f
Chrisman-Snook procedure, 165

Hill-Sachs lesions
arthroscopy of, 2
staple capsulorrhaphy for, 27

Iliotibial band transfer, Ellison procedure
in anterior cruciate ligament repair, 135, 138–142, 138–141f
capsule repair in, 141
dissection procedures, 138–139, 139f
with fibular collateral ligament, 139–140, 140f
incisions for, 138, 138f
in lateral collateral ligament repair, 126–127
in medial collateral ligament repair, 115, 116f
meniscectomy with, 139
with patellar tendon, 140, 141f, 142, 144, 146
techniques of, 138–142, 138–141f
Impingement syndrome of shoulder, 8–18
bicipital tenodesis for, 16–18
    general considerations, 16–17
    techniques of, 17, 17f, 18f

coracoacromial ligament resection for, 8–11
    contraindications to, 9
    general considerations, 8–9
    indications for, 8
    postoperative care and rehabilitation, 10–11
    techniques of, 9–10, 9f, 10f
diagnosis of, 8–9
rehabilitative protocol for, 82–83
    after coracoacromial ligament resection, 10–11
    after rotator cuff repair, 16, 83
rotator cuff repair for, 11–16
    general considerations, 11
    postoperative care and rehabilitation, 16
    techniques of, 11–16, 11–16f
Iontophoresis, 63, 63f

Jumper's knee, 105

Knee injuries
of anterior cruciate ligament. See Anterior cruciate ligament injuries of knee
arthroscopy of. See Arthroscopy of knee injuries
exercises for. See Exercises for knee
extensor mechanism, 105–109
    patellar tendinitis repair of, 105–106, 106f
    patellar tendon rupture repair of, 107–109, 108f, 109f
of lateral collateral ligament. See Lateral collateral ligament injuries of knee
of medial collateral ligament. See Medial collateral ligament injuries of knee
patellar malalignment syndromes, 99–104
    computerized tomography of, 99
    diagnosis of, 99
    general considerations, 99
    postoperative care and rehabilitation for, 104
    surgical treatment of, 100–104, 100–103f
patellar tendinitis
    general considerations, 105
    postoperative care and rehabilitation for, 106
    surgical repair of, 105–106, 106f
patellar tendon rupture, 107–109
    causes of, 107
    general considerations of, 107

Knee injuries (*Cont.*)
  postoperative care and rehabilitation
    for, 109
  surgical repair of, 107–109, 108f,
    109f
  of posterior cruciate ligament. *See* Pos-
    terior cruciate ligament injuries of
    knee
  rehabilitation programs for. *See* Reha-
    bilitation programs for knee
    injuries
  stress testing of, 111, 112

Lachman test, 111, 134
Lateral collateral ligament injuries of
  knee
  acute, repair of, 123–125
    general considerations, 123
    capsule tear in, 124
    cruciate ligaments in, 124
    dissection procedures, 123–124,
      124f
    evaluation prior to, 123
    incisions for, 123, 123f, 124
    peroneal nerve in, 124, 124f, 125
    popliteus tendon in, 124, 124f
    postoperative care and rehabilitation,
      125
    techniques of, 123–125, 123–125f
  cause of, 123
  chronic, repair of, 123–125
    evaluation prior to, 125
    extra-articular repairs, 125–126
    general considerations, 125–126
    iliotibial band transfer in, 126
    intra-articular reconstruction, 125,
      126, 126f
    postoperative care and rehabilitation,
      127
    techniques of, 126–127, 126f, 127f
  evaluation of
    for acute injuries, 123
    for chronic injuries, 125
  rehabilitation programs for
    acute injuries, 125
    chronic injuries, 127
    protocols for, 189
Lateral epicondyle of elbow
  in arthroscopy, 41
  in debridement of loose bodies, 46,
    47f
  inflammation of, 43
  release of, 43–45
    anesthesia for, 43
    dissection procedures, 43–44, 43–
      44f
    excision of degenerative area in, 44,
      44f
    general considerations, 43
    indications for, 43
    postoperative care and rehabilitation
      for, 45

techniques of, 43–44, 43–45f
Lateral ligament injuries of ankle
  Brostrom reconstruction procedure for,
    162–165
    general considerations, 162
    postoperative care and rehabilitation
      for, 165
    techniques of, 162–165, 162–165,
      163–165f
  Chrisman-Snook reconstruction proce-
    dure for, 165–169
    general considerations, 165
    postoperative care and rehabilitation,
      169
    techniques of, 166–168, 166–169f

Medial collateral ligament injuries of
  knee
  acute, repair of, 111–118
    anterior cruciate ligament in, 111,
      114–115, 117f
    capsule tear in, 117–118, 117f
    dissection procedures, 112–114,
      113f, 114f
    general considerations, 111–112
    grafting procedures, 114–118, 115–
      117f
    iliotibial band transfer in, 115, 116f
    incisions for, 112, 112f
    pes anserinus tendons in, 114, 114f,
      118
    posterior cruciate ligament in, 111,
      115–117, 116f, 117f
    postoperative care and rehabilitation
      for, 118
    techniques of, 112–118, 112–118f
    with tibial avulsion, 115
    evaluation prior to, 111–112
  cause of, 111
  chronic, repair of, 119–121
    anterior cruciate ligament in, 119,
      120
    dissection procedures, 119–120,
      119f
    evaluation prior to, 119
    general considerations, 119
    incisions for, 119
    meniscal tear removal in, 120
    Nicholas procedure, 119
    postoperative care and rehabilitation,
      120–121
    techniques of, 119–120, 119–121f
  evaluation of
    for acute injuries, 111, 112
    for chronic injuries, 119
  rehabilitation programs for, 189
    for acute injuries, 118
    for chronic injuries, 120–121
  sprains, 111
  tears, 111
Medial collateral ligament injuries of
  elbow

general considerations, 49
surgical repair of, 49–52, 49–52f
  incisions for, 49–50, 49–50f
  indications for, 49
  palmaris longus tendon transplant in,
    50–51, 50–51f
  postoperative care and rehabilitation,
    52
  techniques for, 49–52, 49–52f
  ulnar nerve transfer in, 52, 52f
Medial epicondyle of elbow
  in arthroscopy, 41
  in ulnar nerve transfer, 54

Os calcis beak
  Achilles tendon inflammation and rup-
    ture from, 155
  resection of, 157, 158, 158f
Osteochondritis dissecans of talus. *See*
  Talus injuries, osteochondritis
  dissecans

Patellar chondromalacia, 191–192
Patellar malalignment syndrome
  computerized tomography of, 99
  diagnosis of, 99
  general considerations of, 99
  surgical treatment of, 100–104, 100–
    103f
    dissection procedures for, 100–101,
      100f
    incisions for, 100, 100f
    indications for, 99
    postoperative care and rehabilitation,
      104
    for proximal realignment, 101
    tibial tubercle transfer in, 101–103,
      102f
Patellar tendon
  in iliotibial band transfer, 140–141,
    141f
  inflammation of, 105
    from extensor mechanism injuries,
      105
    postoperative care and rehablitiation
      for, 106
    surgical repair of, 105–106, 106f
  intra-articular transfer of
    arthrotomies for, 143, 143f
    dissection procedures for, 142, 142f
    grafting procedures in, 144–146,
      145f, 146f
    with iliotibial band, 142, 144, 146
    incisions for, 142, 142f, 143
    meniscectomy with, 143, 146
    with pes anserinus, 146
    techniques of, 142–147, 142–147f
  in medial collateral ligament repair,
    114, 115, 115f
  rupture of, 107–109
    causes of, 107

postoperative care and rehabilitation
for, 109
surgical repair of, 107–109, 108f,
109f
Peroneal nerve dysfunction, 125
Pes anserinus transfer
in anterior cruciate ligament repair,
135–138
dissection procedures, 135–136, 136f,
137f
with Ellison procedure, 138
incisions for, 135, 135f
in medial collateral ligament repair,
114, 114f, 118, 138
with patellar tendon, 146
saphenous nerve considerations in,
136, 136f
techniques of, 135–138, 135–137f
Phonophoresis, 63, 64f
Posterior cruciate ligament injuries of
knee
acute, repair of
arthroscopy in, 128
avulsion injuries, 129
capsule tear in, 129
dissection procedures, 130, 130f
evaluation of injury prior to, 128
gastrocnemius muscle tendon transfer in, 130–132, 132f, 191
general considerations, 128
incisions for, 128, 129f, 130
with lateral collateral ligament repair, 124
with medial collateral ligament repair, 111, 115–118, 116f, 117f
techniques of, 128–129, 129f
cause of, 128
chronic, repair of
evaluation of injury prior to, 129
general considerations, 129
postoperative care and rehabilitation,
133
techniques of, 130–132, 130–132f
evaluation of
for acute injuries, 111, 128
for chronic injuries, 129
function considerations, 128, 191
rehabilitation programs for, 191

Rehabilitation programs
for ankle injuries, 192–198
advanced phase of, 196–198
goals of, 176, 177–178
immediate postoperative, 176–177
intermediate phase of, 194–196
during immobilization period, 177
incomplete, reinjury due to, 176
physical examination prior to, 178
starting phase of, 192–194
for elbow injuries
advanced phase of, 88–89

Rehabilitation programs (cont.)
after biceps tendon rupture repair,
61
after debridement of loose bodies,
48
deviation exercises in, 86, 86f
extension exercises in, 78, 78f, 87–
88, 88f
finger flexion exercises in, 85–86
flexion exercises in, 78, 78f, 88,
88f
forearm exercises in, 86, 86f, 88
intermediate phase of, 85–88
after medial collateral ligament reconstruction, 52
objectives of, 84
after release of lateral epicondyle,
45
starting phase of, 84–85, 85f
strengthening exercises in, 85–87
stretching exercises in, 87
after ulnar nerve transfer, 55
wrist exercises in, 87, 87f
goals of, determination of
for lower extremity, 177–178
for upper extremity, 62
for knee injuries, 178–192
advanced phase of, 187–188
after anterior cruciate ligament repair, 189–190, 190f
calf exercises, 182–183, 182f, 185–
186, 186f, 187f
after collateral ligament repair, 189
competitive retraining, 188
controlled jogging, 188
Cybex testing in, 187, 187f, 188
development of, 177–178
free weights in, 183–184, 186
gait analysis in, 178
gastrocnemius stretching exercises,
183, 183f
goals of, 176, 177–178
hamstring curls, 184, 185f
hamstring-setting exercises, 181–
182, 182f
hip abduction exercises, 179, 179f,
181, 184, 185f
hip adduction exercises, 180–181,
180f, 184, 185f
hip extension exercises, 180, 180f,
181, 184
hip flexion exercises, 179, 181, 184
home programs, 184, 186, 188
immediate postoperative, 176–177
during immobilization period, 177
incomplete, reinjury due to, 176
intermediate phase of, 184–187
for nonimmobilized portions of
body, 177
Orthotron usage, 187
pain tolerance in, 178
after patellar chondromalacia repair,
191–192

Rehabilitation programs (cont.)
physical examination prior to, 178
after posterior cruciate ligament repair, 191
quadriceps resistive exercises, 184–
185, 186f
quadriceps-setting exercises, 181,
181f
short-arc quadriceps exercises, 181,
182f
starting phase of, 178–184
step-up exercises, 185–186, 186f
straight-leg raise exercises, 181,
181f
stretching exercises, 183, 183f
tilt-board exercises, 184, 184f
toe-raise exercises, 182–183, 182f,
186, 187f
towel-stretch exercises, 183, 183f
wall-slide exercises, 178, 179f, 184
warmup exercises, 178, 179f, 184,
184f
for shoulder injuries
abduction exercises in, 73–75, 73f,
74f, 79, 80f, 81f
adduction exercises in, 77, 77f
advanced phase of, 79–82
anterior capsule stretching exercises
in, 70–71, 70f, 71f
after anterior reconstruction, 30,
83–84
basic protocol for, 62–82
after capsulorrhaphy, anterior staple,
30, 83
after coracoacromial ligament resection, 10–11
elbow flexion and extension exercises in, 78, 78f
extension exercises in, 70, 70f, 77–
78, 78f
flexion exercises in, 73, 73f
home exercises, 69, 79
for impingement syndrome, 82–83
inferior capsule stretching exercises
in, 71, 72f
intermediate phase of, 70–79
isometric exercises in, 69, 69f
joint mobilization in, 68, 68f
after modified Bristow reconstruction, 27, 83
objectives of, 62
pendulum exercises in, 64–66, 65f
posterior capsule stretching exercises
in, 72, 72f
after posterior reconstruction, 36
progressive resistance exercises in,
72–73
rotational stretching exercises, 63–
64, 65f
external, 75–76, 75f
internal, 76, 76f
after rotator cuff repair, 16, 83
saw exercises in, 64, 65f

Rehabilitation programs (*cont.*)
  shrug exercises in, 66, 66f, 77
  special protocols for, 82–84
  starting phase of, 62–69
  stretching exercises in, 63–64, 65f,
    70–72, 70–72f
  throwing exercises in, 81–82
  treatment of pain in, 63, 63f, 64f
  wall slide exercises in, 66–67, 66f
  wand exercises in, 67, 67f, 68f
  warm-up exercises in, 62–63, 63f
Rotator cuff
  arthroscopy of, 2, 4
  rupture of, repair of, 11–16, 11–16f
    acromioplasty for, 13, 13f
    postoperative care and rehabilitation
      of, 16, 83
    reapproximation of deltoid in, 12,
      14–16, 16f
    soft tissue graft for, 14, 15f

Shoulder injuries
  anterior reconstruction for, 20–31
    via Bristow procedure, modified.
      See Bristow procedure, modified
    via staple capsulorrhaphy. *See* Staple
      capsulorrhaphy of shoulder,
      anterior
  arthroscopy of. *See* Arthroscopy of
    shoulder injuries
  diagnosis of, 20, 32
  exercises for. *See* Exercises for
    shoulder
  impingement syndrome of. *See* Im-
    pingement syndrome of shoulder
  posterior reconstruction for, 32–37
    general considerations, 32
    indications for, 32

  postoperative care and rehabilitation
    for, 36, 84
  techniques of, 32–36, 33–37f
  rehabilitation programs for. *See* Re-
    habilitation programs for shoulder
    injuries
  staple capsulorrhaphy for. *See* Staple
    capsulorrhaphy of shoulder
Staple capsulorrhaphy of shoulder ante-
    rior, 27–30
  general considerations, 27
  indications for, 27
  postoperative care and rehabilitation
    for, 30, 83
  techniques of, 27–30, 28–30f
  posterior, 32–37
    for Bankart lesion, 34
    dissection procedures, 32–34, 33–
      35f
    general considerations, 32
    indications and contraindications for,
      32
    patient position for, 32
    postoperative care and rehabilitation
      for, 36, 84
    techniques of, 32–36, 33–37f
Subscapularis muscle and tendon
  arthroscopy of, 4, 5f, 6f
  in modified Bristow procedure, 23
  in staple capsulorrhaphy, 27, 28f

Talocalcaneal ligament reconstruction,
    165, 165f
Talofibular ligament reconstruction
  Brostrom procedure for, 162–165,
    163f, 164f
  Chrisman-Snook procedure for, 165,
    166, 168
Talus injuries

  osteochondral fracture, 171
  osteochrondritis dissecans
    dissection procedures for localization
      of, 171–172, 172f
    excision of lesions of, 172–173,
      173f
    general considerations, 171
    malleolus osteotomy for excision of
      lesions of, 173, 174f
    postoperative care and rehabilitation
      for, 173
    surgical treatment of, 171–173,
      171–174f
Tibiofibular ligament reconstruction
  Brostrom procedure for, 162, 163f
  Chrisman-Snook procedure for, 166
Transcutaneous electrical stimulation, 63

Ulnar collateral ligament injuries of el-
    bow, 49
Ulnar nerve
  branches of, 54, 54f
  irritation of, 53
  transfer of
    anesthesia for, 53
    dissection procedures, 53–54, 54f
    general considerations, 53
    incisions for, 53, 53f
    indications for, 53
    intermuscular septum resection for,
      54
    in medial collateral ligament recon-
      struction, 52, 52f
    postoperative care and rehabilitation,
      55
    techniques of, 53–55, 53–55f

Wrist exercises, 85, 85f, 87, 87f